Marijuana Killed My Cancer
and is keeping me cancer free

Marijuana Killed My Cancer and is keeping me cancer free

Step-by-step guide how to kill your cancer with cannabis
The healing miracle of CBD plus THC

Erika M. Karohs Ph.D.

Published by:
Erika M. Karohs Ph.D.

ISBN: 1523752343
ISBN 13: 9781523752348

Disclaimer

The author provides the material in this book "as is" without warranty of any kind, expressed or implied, including, but not limited to the accuracy or completeness of the material or the implied warranties for any particular purpose.

The material is not intended to be, and should not be considered, a substitute for professional and/or medical expert advice. Information in this book is solely for educational purposes about a natural remedy for cancer. It is not intended as an alternative to medical diagnosis or treatment.

The author made the greatest effort to offer accurate information regarding the subject matter and to be current as of the time it was written. However, research into medical cannabis is ongoing and new knowledge is constantly evolving. Readers should therefore always check the most up-to-date published information, including dosage information and safety regulations.

The author does not accept, and expressly disclaims, any responsibility or any liability, for loss, or risk, or damage that may be claimed or incurred as a result of the use and/or application of any of the contents of this book.

By reading this book or using the information provided, you agree that there is no recourse available regarding liability. If you do not agree, please do not read further. Reading or using the information contained herein constitutes agreement with the stated liability conditions.

If you are suffering from any serious malady, before doing anything, you should seek professional medical attention. Do not delay seeking medical advice, or discontinue medical treatment because of information in this book.

Before starting any changes in your life style, or in using medication or supplements, consult with your doctor.

Do not do anything illegal!

Statements in this book have not been evaluated by the Food and Drug Administration (FDA).

(For confidentiality reasons, the personal names of patients mentioned in this book have been changed to protect the innocent victims of cancer. All the testimonial letters are in my files.)

Foreword

My son Michael asked me to write this book because it is something he wishes he could have read three years ago when he was diagnosed with cancer. Below is his story in his own words.

I am a cancer survivor. I am telling my story for you, my fellow cancer patients, because I was once in your shoes. I want to spare you the shock, the fear, the desperation, the agony, the helplessness, the confusion, and the desperate search for solutions that I went through. Believe me, if you are diagnosed with cancer, I know how exactly how you feel.

But let me also tell you another thing that nobody told me when I was diagnosed with this devastating disease:

Cancer can be cured! Yes. Cancer can be cured, often inexpensively and with few or no side effects, and even without patients having to leave home.

Cannabis CAN cure cancer.

Chemotherapy, long considered the most effective cancer treatment, may actually backfire. Recent studies have shown that this aggressive treatment severely damages healthy cells and triggers them to release a protein WNT16B that actually fuels tumor growth. Once secreted, this protein interacts with nearby tumor cells. It causes them to grow and resist further treatment; instead of killing them, it actually boosts cancer cell survival. Rates of tumor cell reproduction have been shown to accelerate between treatments, thereby killing patients more quickly.

Researchers made these findings while seeking to explain why cancer cells are so resilient inside the human body when they are easy to kill in the lab. "The increase in WNT16B was completely unexpected," said co-author Peter Nelson of the Fred Hutchinson Cancer Research Center in Seattle.

The researchers said they confirmed their findings with breast and ovarian cancer tumors.

Cannabis is the only therapy that is completely anti-cancer. It kills cancer in a variety of ways, while at the same time promoting the development of new, healthy cells. And it kills cancer cells without damaging side effects. Cannabis always helps the body; it never assaults it, as is so often the case with chemotherapy and other conventional treatments.

The results of thousands of studies have shown that cannabis may well be the single most powerful medicine for curing cancer.

I know because I cured myself with cannabis. Cancer-stricken friends with whom I have shared the information were also healed. So were people in our cancer support group. Using this book as a guide you too can learn how to create your own cannabis healing miracle.

From a patient's wife:
Jim's oncologist just reviewed his blood tests and said that Jim is in Remission!!!!!!! WOW. From stage 4 lymphoma and leukemia!!! I k.n.o.w it is the oil. His lymph nodes are all back to normal size. The blood tests do not show the signs of the cancer anymore. Amazing!

From a patient:
Mike, I continue to be blessed with getting a bit better every day...I went to the oncologist on the 6th. I feel so wonderful that he has seen fit to keep me off chemo.
Last year, after the first surgery, they put me in a chemo chair three days after I was out of the hospital! That's when they told me, I would never be fully cured...and now they can no longer find the cancer.
Amy (March 15, 2015)

Yes, yes, I know there are many people out there who do not want to believe this, who choose not to believe it, who obsessively argue against it, and refuse to even consider anything else. Fine.

In all fairness, I must admit that I don't care a whit about them, their beliefs, their fanaticism, their prejudice—or their pocketbooks. (Yes, cancer is a gravy train for many. Did you know that the average cancer patient generates $1.3 million dollars in revenue for the cancer industry?) But this book is not written for them. It is written for people who are scared out of their minds because they feel they have been given a death sentence and have nowhere to turn.

If you are a cancer patient you made a smart decision to select this book. It is chockfull of information how to kill your cancer. It explains everything, along with step-by-step instructions. But remember, things will not happen automatically. You have to be committed to do your part, and you have to be willing to follow through. A hit and miss program will not work. Just reading the book is of no value. If you do start let nothing and no one interfere.

If you want – REALLY want – to heal, and stay healthy, all you have to do is start your own cannabis healing program and stick with it!

So what are you waiting for? Go! START RIGHT NOW!

Table of Contents

My personal story

Cancer hits most people with little or no warning, rapidly devastating and destroying their lives. Few other diseases cause so much heartbreak, fear, depression, grief and suffering as does cancer.

Sherwin Nuland wrote in his book *How We Die,* "[cancer] pursues a continuous, uninhibited, circumferential, barn-burning expedition of destructiveness, in which it heeds no rules, follows no commands, [and] explodes all resistance in a homicidal riot of destructiveness."[1]

I have experienced the sense of dread and fear that cancer instills; I am a cancer survivor, and this is my story.

On 27 November 2012 I was rushed to Emergency. I nearly died during the 10-minute ride to the hospital and had to be resuscitated by the paramedics.

At the hospital I was put on life support, hydrating fluids, and intravenous feeding. Before starting tests, doctors were already 99% sure that I had colon cancer. I had lost nearly 100 pounds within a few months and had excruciating abdominal pains.

It took two weeks until I was strong enough to have a chance of surviving the first operation—a colostomy procedure. One week later a very large, very aggressive tumor was removed.

To the doctors' surprise the pathology report showed that my cancer was actually Hodgkin's lymphoma rather than colon cancer. The exact diagnosis was:

Large cell lymphoma, unspecified site, extranodal and solid organ sites
Nausea with vomiting

---

1 Sherwin Nuland, How We Die, Alfred A Knopf, New York, 1994, p. 207.

Neutropenia unspecified
Encounter for antineoplastic chemotherapy

Hodgkin's lymphoma (HL) is one of the most frequent lymphomas in the Western world. Although the majority of HL cases at any clinical stage have a good prognosis under adequate therapy, many patients still develop a highly mortal relapse.

I was fortunate that an experienced and skilled surgeon was able to remove the entire tumor intact. I also owe thanks to my caring and knowledgeable oncologist. Without those doctors and my wonderful nurses, I probably would not have survived. Still, I lost my colon and part of the small intestines, and I still have a colostomy.

After surgery I was informed that without follow-up treatment with chemotherapy and possibly radiation this very aggressive kind of cancer was almost certain to kill me.

Consequently, three months after surgery I was put on five lymphoma-specific chemo drugs. Follow-up with radiation was being considered.

During chemotherapy sessions and support group meetings I learned that most patients go the conventional route: surgery (cutting out any malignant mass), chemo (administering not quite fatal doses of strong poisons) and radiation (burning out diseased tissues). In other words, tumors are cut out, poisoned, or burned. These seem to be the accepted methods for treating cancer. Never mind that they are traumatic, debilitating, and terrifying to the patients, and that after a temporary remission cancer often recurs, either in the same organ, or in other parts of the body. And then the cycle begins anew until the patient is too weak to endure further treatment. Ironically, most cancer deaths occur while patients are under treatment, which is so debilitating that ultimately the patient dies.

The Envita cancer clinic in Scottsdale Arizona reports:

"The data has now become clear that after initial chemotherapy fails, as many as 95% of cancer patients will not respond to the next suggested drug by conventional methods."[2]

2 Www.envita.com/cancer/cancer-treatment-the-2nd-opinion-that-is-saving-lives

Cancer drugs, pushed by many pharmaceutical companies as the only "scientific" method beside chemotherapy, have been shown to often enhance cancer and kill patients more quickly. According to a study in the January 2015 issue of "Cancer Cell, "cancer drugs sold at exorbitant prices to cancer patients are not only ineffective but also hazardous. While they temporarily reduce tumor size, they subsequently cause tumors to metastasize. The tumors come back much stronger and grow much larger than their original size."

"Whatever manipulations we're doing to tumors can inadvertently do something to increase the tumor numbers to become more metastatic, which is what kills patients at the end of the day," lamented study author Dr. Raghu Kalluri.

Why then are doctors continuing this kind of treatment? Why don't they tell patients about alternative options? Why? The reason behind it is pretty obvious. It is M-O-N-E-Y ! According to "Health Impact News," the typical new cancer drug coming on the market in 2005 cost about $4,500 per month; since 2010 the median price has been around $10,000. In 2015, two of the new cancer drugs cost more than $35,000 each per month of treatment.

The more I thought about this, the more I realized this route was not for me.

I methodically searched for alternative treatments but most of what I found was snake oil information—dishonest people trying to sell questionable treatments to vulnerable patients. While cancer patients are facing some of the most difficult decisions in their lives, suffering through painful treatments, not to mention the fear that their cancer will kill them, unscrupulous people are trying to peddle so-called "miracle cures," often with fancy sales pitches.

Ever since I was diagnosed I had, in the back of my mind, the idea that I should look into medical cannabis, particularly cannabis oil. I remembered seeing YouTube videos and reading articles about people having cured themselves from various cancers without negative side effects. My belief was reinforced when a hospital nurse whispered into my ear: "You better seek alternative treatment."

Once I started searching, I found a wealth of information in books, articles, on YouTube, and on the Internet. Over and over, I read about people curing themselves with cannabis, often after they had been given up as incurable by the medical establishment.

PubMed (http://www.ncbi.nlm.nih.gov/pubmed/), a government website, lists thousands of marijuana articles. Of course, many of them are "anti-pot"; but there is also a surprising amount of information about marijuana as cancer treatment and about various cannabis therapies.

The information was mind-blowing: cannabis inhibiting tumor growth, marijuana preventing lung cancer, cannabis antitumor effect with breast cancer, cannabidiol (CBD) inducing apoptosis (self-killing) in leukemia cells, anti-cancer activity in human melanoma cells, cannabis fighting pancreatic cancer, and cannabis lowering the incidence of diabetes or delaying the onset of the disease.

Researchers at the California Medical Center Research Institute combined the non-psychoactive cannabis compound CBD (cannabidiol) with delta-9-tretrahydrocannabinol (Δ9-THC), the primary psychoactive ingredient in cannabis, to treat brain cancer. They found that the combination boosts the inhibitory effects of Δ9-THC on glioblastoma, the most common and aggressive form of brain tumor.

I read that Delta-9-THC effectively lowered spleen inflammation linked to leukemia, and that bone marrow treated with delta-8-THC and delta-9-THC showed resistance to cancer.

Preliminary studies have shown that cannabis may also have therapeutic uses for migraines, fibromyalgia, asthma, and epilepsy, Tourette syndrome, PDST and MRSA. Cannabis may also protect people from osteoporosis later in life.

I learned that the use of cannabis as medicine is not a new concept at all. During the 1800's until 1937, pharmaceutical companies themselves produced many cannabis-based compounds. Also, cannabis has been used as medicine by many cultures for centuries. In India and China the history of medicinal cannabis use dates back thousands of years.

But although there was an abundance of information, to my dismay I found nothing about cannabis curing lymphoma.

Then came the day that changed my life.

I had just started another search when the headline blazed across the screen: "Cannabis May Provide Treatment for Hodgkin's Lymphoma."

(http://thejointblog.com/cannabis-may-provide-treatment-hodgkin-lymphoma/).

Researchers at the German universities of Leipzig and Halle were excited to find cannabinoid receptors[3] as a feature of Hodgkin's lymphoma. They concluded, "Given that cannabis serves as a direct and natural agonist to our body's cannabinoid receptors, cannabis may provide an ideal treatment for this cancer, which is responsible for hundreds of deaths each year according to the American Cancer Society."

After reading and re-reading this study, I decided to forego all further conventional treatments and rely only on cannabis to keep me cancer free.[4]

I secured a legally required "Therapeutic Cannabis Recommendation" and started treating myself with cannabis. Several months later doctors confirmed that I was cancer free.

In December 2014, almost two years after the original diagnosis, I was officially declared cured. Doctors assured me that no further treatment was needed, and that there was very little chance that my cancer would ever return.

Before delving further into my incredible journey from cancer diagnosis to cure, an explanation about the marvelous endocannabinoid system and the amazing endocannabinoids seems indicated. Chances are, you've never heard of either one of them. Few people have—including doctors.

---

3 Cannabinoid receptors are explained in the next chapter "The Endocannabinoid System".

4 Cannabis and marijuana both have the same meaning. Cannabis is the botanical name for the plant genus and includes the three varieties cannabis sativa, cannabis indica, and cannabis ruderalis. This book uses the term cannabis to refer to medical marijuana. Since there is no plant named "marijuana," from a botanical point of view, cannabis is the correct term.

The Endocannabinoid System—We Need It for Good Health

Surprising as this may sound but our bodies actually produce substances that are similar to those found in the cannabis plant. They are called endogenous cannabinoids or for short, endocannabinoids. Endocannabinoids are regulated by the Endocannabinoid System (EC), which was first described in 1998 by Israeli scientists Shimon Ben-Shabat and Raphael Mechoulam.

The endocannabinoid system is not unique to the human species. Rather, research has shown that it is present in humans and animals—fish, reptiles, earthworms, leeches, amphibians, slugs, birds and mammals—except insects. Researchers believe that the endocannabinoid system has existed in living organisms for 500 million years.

Actually, mother's milk provides endocannabinoids to the infant. As we mature we produce our own, albeit not always adequately.

The endocannabinoid system consists of a series of receptors, which are found throughout the body: in the brain, organs, connective tissues, glands, and immune cells, in the cardiovascular system, the gastrointestinal and the urinary tract. The two main receptors that have so far been identified are CB1 and CB2. CB1 receptors are primarily found in the brain, but they are also present in adipose tissue (fat) as well as in the stomach, lungs, liver, and in the male and female reproductive organs. CB2 receptors are present in the gut, spleen, liver, heart, kidneys, bones, blood vessels, lymph cells, endocrine glands, and in the reproductive organs.

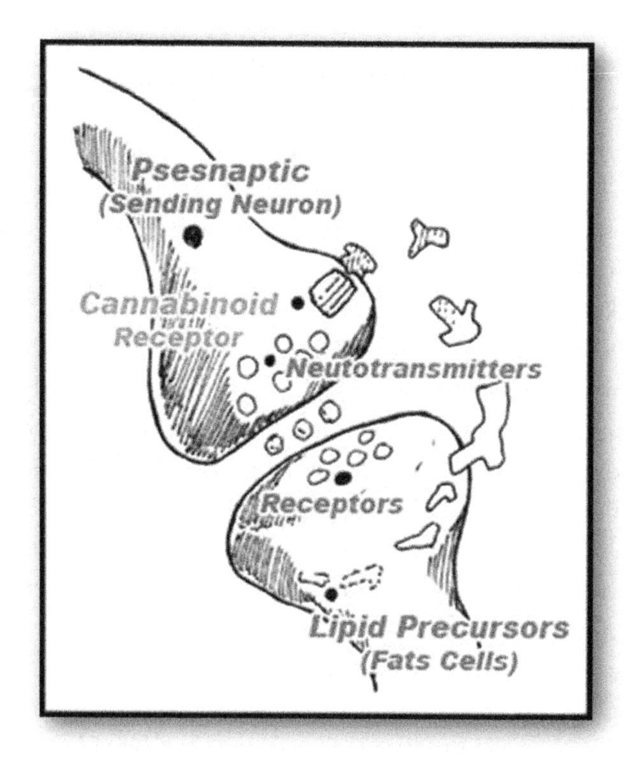

Many tissues contain both CB1 and CB2 receptors, each linked to a different action in the body. Researchers speculate there may be a third cannabinoid receptor waiting to be discovered.

In each part of the body, cannabinoids perform different tasks. The cannabinoids emit signals to which the receptors respond. But the overall goal is always the same: homeostasis—the maintenance of a stable internal environment despite fluctuations in the external environment. According to Dr. Mechoulam, "There is barely a biological, physiological system in our bodies in which the endocannabinoids do not participate."

Research seems to point more and more to the fact that a properly functioning endocannabinoid system is necessary for good health and that deficient cannabinoid levels may be the underlying cause of numerous conditions that can be alleviated by cannabis.

Interestingly, Dr. Robert Melamede, former Biology Department chair and current Professor at the University of Colorado–Colorado Springs, holds the belief that endocannabinoids can inhibit the aging process. "Nobody dies from getting old," he explained. "People die from age-related illnesses." He speculates that cannabinoids are essential nutrients with the ability to minimize age-related illnesses like cancer, cardiovascular disease, Alzheimer's, autoimmune diseases, or skeletal diseases like osteoporosis. Pretty exciting stuff, isn't it?

But while our bodies make their own cannabinoids, they produce only small amounts, sufficient to maintain the body, but not enough to overcome chronic stress, illness, injury, or malnutrition. If the body is in chronic disease or stress mode, the endocannabinoid system can fall behind and lose control of compromised systems. It is here that plant cannabinoids, usually called "phytocannabinoids," can pitch in to supercharge the body's endocannabinoid system. In other words, phytocannabinoids are the perfect remedy for a defunct endocannabinoid system.

How do they work? Glad you asked.

CB receptors are programmed to respond to both the endocannabinoids that our bodies normally produce and to phytocannabinoids, which are plant based, like tetrahydrocannabinol (THC) and cannabidiol (CBD). Research has shown that surprisingly, human cannabinoid receptors seem to have a greater affinity for plant cannabinoids than for those produced within the body itself. As soon as the plant cannabis molecules make contact with the body, there seems to be automatic recognition. Even small doses of plant cannabinoids can signal the body to make more endocannabinoids and build more cannabinoid receptors.

While drug warriors keep trying to persuade us that marijuana is dangerous, a vast amount of evidence is showing the effectiveness of cannabinoids in treating cancer. From brain cancer to lung cancer and breast cancer, the findings are the same: cannabis kills cancer. Most exciting is the fact that cannabinoids not only suppress the survival, growth and spread of cancer cells, but they actually kill cancer in a variety of ways:

- Triggering cell death, through a mechanism called apoptosis (programmed cell death). Apoptosis is originally a Greek term, meaning "the falling away of leaves." Today it is used to describe the natural death process of cells. Cannabinoids selectively trigger the death of malignant cells while leaving healthy cells alone. One of the greatest problem with conventional cancer therapy is that it destroys tumor as well as healthy cells, resulting in nausea, anemia, and hair loss, as intestinal and hair cells are destroyed along with cancer cells. Research suggests that cannabinoid compounds could be developed into a much safer and more effective chemotherapy agent.

- Stopping cells from dividing.
- Preventing formation of new blood vessels by tumors (anti-angiogenesis).
- Reducing the chances of cancer cells spreading through the body, by stopping cells from moving or invading neighboring tissue (anti-metastatic effect).
- Speeding up autophagy (self-eating). This process devours unnecessary or abnormal components within a cell. It keeps healthy cells alive, while at the same time it has a deadly effect on unhealthy cells, such as tumor cells. Tumor cells are ordered to consume themselves in a programmed form of cellular suicide.

And, as if this were not enough, cannabis seems to have potent anti-inflammatory mechanisms that keep healthy cells from turning malignant in the first place. And, in contrast to traditional treatments, cannabis destroys cancerous cells while sparing the surrounding healthy cells and perhaps even protecting them.

The discovery of the endocannabinoid system has greatly changed man's entire understanding of cannabis and its effect. Nearly everything we had been taught since the beginning of the anti-marijuana campaign in the 1930's has been wrong. Instead of the dangerously intoxicating "devil's weed" cannabis is one of the most nourishing, healing plants that can greatly improve and even prolong life.

Conversely, evidence suggests that blocking endocannabinoid receptor activity can have disastrous results on the body. Several years ago, the international pharmaceutical company Sanofi-Aventis developed the drug Rimonabant. The drug blocked CB1 receptor activity, which, it was hoped, would suppress appetite and prevent compulsive eating. The European Medicines Agency EMEA approved Rimonabant in Europe in 2006 as an over-the-counter drug. The U.S. Food and Drug Administration denied approval due to concerns about possible side effects.

In 2008, the EMEA decided to re-evaluate the drug's benefits and side effects. An alarming number of users experienced worrisome symptoms like anxiety, depression, panic attacks, and frequent falls leading to concussions, traffic accidents, and other injuries. Others showed gastrointestinal problems. There appeared to be increases in such illnesses as Alzheimer's, Parkinson's disease, and Huntington's disease. A study at the University of Texas in 2008 found that CB1-blocked mice had increased numbers of colon polyps. It became obvious that cannabis and Rimonabant had opposite effects on the likelihood of colon cancer.

The EMEA eventually revoked its approval of Rimonabant, which today is forbidden in Europe and the U.S. It is still peddled over the Internet to unsuspecting customers by Indian pharmaceutical companies.

For decades, people have been brainwashed into thinking negatively about marijuana; thus it is hard for them to believe that cannabis is actually a beneficial and health-giving plant. But as research continues and more and more is known, it is becoming quite clear that cannabis is healthy rather than harmful.

There can no longer be any doubt that using cannabis is good for us. An adequate endocannabinoid supply is vital to keeping our bodies in optimum health and providing a sense of happiness and calm. Conversely, endocannabinoid deficiency has a deleterious effect on mental and physical wellbeing. This it is supported more and more by solid, peer-reviewed clinical and scientific data from around the world.

Chronic pain patients who use herbal cannabis daily for one-year report reduced discomfort and increased quality of life compared to controls, and did not experience the risk of serious side effects according to clinical data published in the "Journal of Pain."

Ethan Russo, M.D., a famous cannabinoid researcher, speaks of an actual "Clinical Endocannabinoid Deficiency" syndrome. He theorizes that many hard-to-treat diseases may be related to endocannabinoid deficiency and may be suitably treated with cannabinoid medicines.

The Cannabis Plant

There are hundreds of different cannabis strains. Although they are all genetically cannabis, they come in different kinds, shapes, and sizes. Likewise, they all show varying components, aromas, yields, genetics, and effects.

The two most major types are Cannabis Sativa and Cannabis Indica. The third major but somewhat lesser known type is Cannabis Ruderalis.

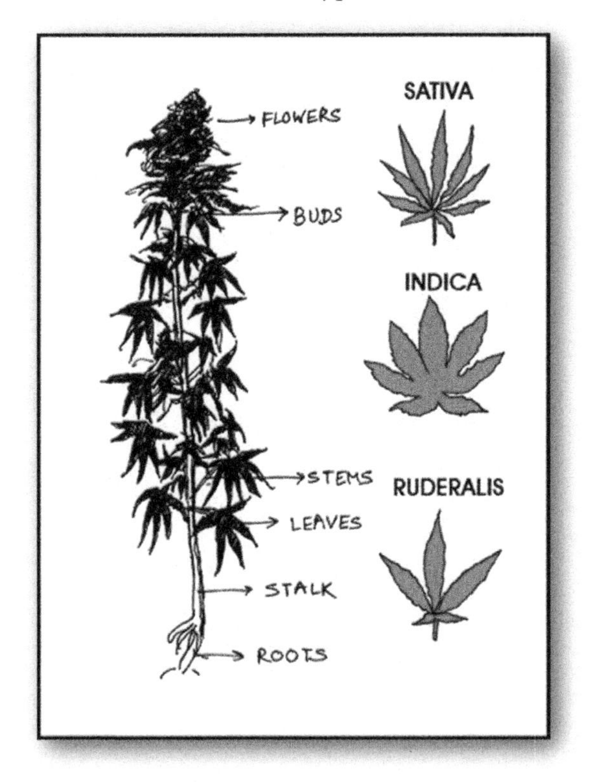

Cannabis sativa

Cannabis sativa strains were officially classified in 1753 in the first edition of *Species Platarum* ("The Species of Plants") by Carolus Linnaeus, a Swedish botanist, zoologist, and taxonomist, also called the "Father of Botany." The word "sativa" comes from the Latin word for "cultivated."

Sativa strains originate from the equatorial regions where daylight hours do not fluctuate in the same way as they do in other regions of the world. There, sativa plants are taking advantage of longer daylight hours with lengthier growing and flowering times. Once flowering has begun, plants can take anywhere from 10 to 16 weeks to fully mature. A positive side effect of the long maturation time is a higher yield. Sativas have long been the most popular variety.

Sativas are the largest of the three varieties and can reach a height in excess of 20 feet (6.1 meters) in one growing season. They are easy to identify because of their long, spindly, serrated leaves. The coloration of the leaves ranges from bright green to almost blackish green. They can display up to thirteen leaflets.

Sativa plants tend to have a higher concentration of THC and relatively low levels of CBD.[5]

Popular sativa strains include Super Silver Haze, Super Lemon Haze, Durban, Blue Dream, and White Widow.

Because of their size and lengthy maturation time sativas had to take a backseat in the minds of many indoor cultivators until finally, shrewd growers crossed them with indica strains. In the hybridized varieties indica genes limit sativa growth while conversely, the influence of sativa makes the indica strains grow taller. Today, there are many sativa/indica hybrids available for indoor cultivation. This allows growers the choice of plants with various desired characteristics and components. The various hybrids will grow and mature in relationship to the sativa/indica percentage they are containing.

---

5 See the following chapter "THC versus CBD" for a detailed explanation.

Cannabis Indica

Cannabis Indica received its name in 1783 from Jean-Baptiste Lamarck, a French Naturalist. He asserted that the European Cannabis Sativa plant is different from those found in India; he therefore added the name *indica* to differentiate between the species. Cannabis indica was introduced to the United States during the 1970's.

The cannabis indica variety originates from subtropical regions such as Pakistan, Afghanistan, Northern India, Kashmir, and Nepal. Because in these areas daylight fluctuates more than in the equatorial regions, indica plants have a different growing pattern than their sativa counterparts. Once plants have reached their ideal height, they put all their energy into producing flowers, using the available daylight hours as best they can. Because of the plants urgency to flower, the indica variety has a much shorter maturation time.

Indicas are short, dense plants that grow small and bushy. Some people describe them as "squat." Outdoors they seldom reach heights of more than 7 feet (2.1 meters). Their leaves are wider and shorter than sativa leaves; they are also more rounded and frequently show a marble pattern. They typically have seven to nine leaflets.

Indica leaves are often darker than any of the other varieties. The buds, too, are different from those of the sativa strains. Whereas sativas have long, sausage-shaped flowers the indica buds are wider.

Indica strains typically have a much higher CBD content than sativas. Because the CBD effect is usually more physical, it is often used as pain reliever and relaxant.

Cannabis indica grows much more quickly than sativa and has a shorter flowering time. The shorter maturation time and the plants' much smaller stature makes the indica variety especially popular with indoor growers.

The most popular Indica strains currently include Afghani, Kosher Kush, Big Bud, and Purple Kush.

Cannabis Ruderalis

The *Cannabis Ruderalis* variety is not nearly as popular as the sativa and indica strains. It was named in 1924 by Russian botanist Janischewski who named it *Ruderalis*, which is the Russian word for "ruderal plant." (*Ruderal* plant species are the ones that are first to inhabit devastated lands, like those damaged after an earthquake or through human activities.)

Ruderalis is an extremely hardy, harsh, non-domesticated plant, which grows like a weed in the colder regions of the world, most often in China and Russia.

Ruderalis contains virtually no THC and has long been ignored by the cannabis community due to the species' inability to get people high. But it is extremely rich in CBD. Actually, ruderalis displays a chemical profile similar to hemp.

The main feature of ruderalis is that it is auto-flowering. This means it needs far less care than sativas and indicas. Ruderalis grows fast and well by itself.

The ruderalis plants are generally short and usually only grow to about 2 feet tall. They produce small leaves that may contain from five to thirteen leaflets. The plant usually produces only a few side branches.

Of late, savvy growers have realized that the auto-flowering capacity of the ruderalis plant could be of great benefit to indoor growing. By crossing indica plants with ruderalis, they created small, manageable plants, which do not need a change in the light cycle to start them flowering. This is a huge advantage to novice growers. A crop can be planted and maintained with little effort. After harvest, a new crop can be planted immediately because flowering will occur according to growing time rather than seasonal changes.

The lowdown on hybrids

Most cannabis seeds and medicines today are from hybrids. "Hybrid" means crossbreeding different species of plants together. Sativas, indicas and ruderalis strains are all capable of crossbreeding. This allows the grower to manipulate plant characteristics and even create new hybrid strains with emphasis upon the more desirable medicinal characteristics.

Examples of hybrid strains are:

- indica x sativa
- indica x indica
- sativa x sativa
- sativa x indica
- indica x ruderalis
- sativa x ruderalis

Hybrids containing ruderalis are typically more resistant to insect infestation and disease. Most often, they also have a higher CBD content.

There can also be numerous three- and four-way hybrids. Many of these have shown strong medical properties because they bring additional ingredients into the mix.

Occasionally, hybrids can produce some really strange mutations, some of them being worthless, and some of them being incredibly useful and interesting.

For example, some male hybrid plants seem to develop fully and look absolutely perfect; yet they are incapable of producing any pollens whatsoever. They are totally useless and have to be discarded.

THC versus CBD

Cannabis plants can exhibit wide variations in the quantity and type of cannabinoids they produce. Strains for recreational use are mostly bred for their high THC content, while medicinal strains are typically bred for high CBD content.

Initially, it was assumed that CBD preceded THC. Nowadays, information about cannabinoids is much more extensive than in the past. We now know that THC and CBD are produced independently of each other.

So far, at least 85 cannabinoids have been identified. The better-known ones are:

- THC (Tetrahydrocannabinol)
- CBD Cannabidiol
- CBG Cannabigerol
- CBN Cannabinol
- CBC Cannabichromene
- CBDV Cannabidivarin
- CBGMCannabigerolMonomethyl Ether
- THCV Tetrahydrocannabivarin.

Although none of these other cannabinoids have the same recognition as THC and CBD, many of them appear to have powerful therapeutic effects on various parts of the body.

Tetrahydrocannabinol (THC)

THC is almost certainly the most popular cannabinoid. Because of its psycho-active effect it is highly sought after by recreational marijuana users.

THC was first isolated in 1964 by Israeli scientists Raphael Mechoulam, Yechiel Gaoni, and the Weizman Institute of Science.

It mimics the action of anandamide, a cannabinoid produced naturally in the body. It creates most of its effect by binding to CB1 receptors in the brain, although it also has an affinity for CB2 receptors.

THC has been found to have several therapeutic applications. It is used for inhibiting cancer cell growth, relieving pain, soothing pain and nausea in people with cancer, stimulating appetite and aiding sleep. Scientists are testing THC's effectiveness in combating multiple sclerosis, Crohn's disease, inflammatory conditions and spinal cord injuries.

When THC stimulates CB1 receptors in the brain, they appear to play an important role in eliminating adverse memories. This is of great benefit in the treatment of PTSD. In fact, the Department of Health and Human Services recently approved a proposal to investigate the potential of cannabis as part of the treatment for veterans with posttraumatic stress disorder.

Cannabidiol (CBD)

Cannabidiol (CBD) is the second leading active ingredient in cannabis; it holds great promise for the treatment of serious medical conditions. Since it is non-psychoactive it does not contribute to a feeling of being "high."

Among the non-psychoactive phytocannabinoids, CBD has aroused the most interest and received the greatest attention.

In Northern California, a group of activists have founded Project CBD, a "not-for profit, educational service dedicated to promoting and publicizing research into the unique medical properties of Cannabidiol (CBD) and other components of the cannabis plant."

Israeli scientist Dr. Raphael Mechoulam identified CBD in 1963, while he was searching for the active ingredient in cannabis. (He discovered THC, the psycho-active ingredient, in 1964.)

CBD has been proven to be effective in the treatment of chronic pain, rheumatoid arthritis, strokes, PDST, cardiovascular disease, seizures, and convulsions. CBD helps in reducing blood sugar levels, reducing inflammation, decreasing risk of artery blockage, slowing bacterial growth, suppressing muscle spasm, and in promoting bone growth and supporting the immune system.

Israeli scientists examined how CBD-rich cannabis extract compared with commercial painkillers and anti-inflammatory drugs. They found that CBD extract exhibited greater anti-inflammatory potency than aspirin.

Scientists at the California Pacific Medical Center found that CBD turns off the genes that cause aggressive cancers like leukemia, pancreatic, lung, ovarian, and brain cancer.

A study published in the journal *Molecular Cancer Therapeutics* reports that CBD stops breast cancer by turning off a gene called Id-1. Cancer cells make more copies of this gene than healthy cells, and this enables cancer to spread through the body.

CBD appears to be at least as strong and anti-inflammatory as Ibuprofen. Its anti-oxidant properties are beneficial in fighting degenerative diseases like Alzheimer's, Parkinson's disease, and autism. In addition, CBD has been shown to assist with general feelings of anxiety.

Research at Temple University has found that CBD may delay the onset of chemotherapy-induced neuropathy, a side effect of some chemotherapy drugs.

CBD is very safe. Patent #66,30,507, held by the U.S. government states the following:

> *"No signs of toxicity or serious side effects have been observed following chronic administration of cannabidiol to healthy volunteers (Cunha et al, Pharmacology 21:175-185, 1980), even in large acute doses of 700/ mg day."*

CBD modifies how THC affects the body, making it less psychoactive and more therapeutic. It promotes a more calming, sedative effect, cutting down on anxiety and memory impairment that many patients find unpleasant and debilitating with regular use of marijuana.

Because CBD is non-psychoactive and strongly therapeutic even in small doses, it is suitable for the treatment of children, the elderly, and anyone who is uncomfortable with a THC "high."

The demand for CBD is steadily growing. More and more cancer patients are learning about the therapeutic effects it has on their disease. Desperate parents are trying to get their hands on CBD-dominant strains for their children with epilepsy and Dravet's Syndrome. This clearly contradicts the charges of drug warriors that medical cannabis users are merely seeking an excuse to get "high."

The legalization of medical cannabis has greatly encouraged research into CBD-rich strains. Regrettably, the current emphasis on CBD-high medicine seems to overshadow the therapeutic role of THC and other cannabis components.

The reality, based upon anecdotal reports, seems to be that cannabis works best as an "entourage" rather than an isolated medicine, and the greatest benefit is gained when THC and CBD work together synergistically—complementing and boosting each compound's positive effects while mitigating negative effects. This synergy elevates the overall effectiveness of the cannabis remedy.

Why THC/CBD Synergy is most effective

Many cancer patients seem to think that CBD is the only active cancer-fighting component in cannabis. But that is a myth.

Both CBD and THC have anti-cancer properties in their own right, but work on different pathways in the body, thereby complementing each other's effects on the same symptoms when administered together.

One of CBD's main benefits is that it boosts THC's effectiveness by lessening its undesirable effects, thus allowing for higher doses of THC to be administered for greater therapeutic effectiveness.

Professor Raphael Mechoulam from Israel, also called the "Father Of Cannabis Research," says that "it is extremely important to know what a person is getting. Not every disease is affected by a same type of marijuana or the same dosage. There are marijuana mixtures with a lot of THC and a little bit of CBD, or vice versa."[6]

TikkunOlam, a Tel Aviv-based company, is concentrating on providing the right type of cannabis to individual patients by providing education on medical cannabis use. They even opened an instruction center.

Tests at the California Pacific Medical Center in San Francisco indicate that best results in breast cancer treatment were obtained when CBD was administered in combination with THC. When present along with THC, CBD prolongs the effects of THC-therapy by inhibiting the breakdown process of THC in the liver. If the THC breakdown is inhibited, its effects persist longer.

Studies at the California Pacific Medical Center in San Francisco are demonstrating that precise combinations of THC and CBD injected into breast and brain tumors can eradicate those cancers in as little as 30 days.

Many problems associated with aging result from the inability of an organism to defend itself against free-radical-induced inflammation and oxidative stress. This provides a fertile ground for the spread of neurodegenerative and other age-related illnesses. Cardiovascular, autoimmune, neurological disorders, cancers, and the aging process itself all have free radicals as a causative agent. A combination of CBD and THC can act as potent anti-oxidant that diminishes the negative effects of oxygen free radicals.

By binding up free radicals, the antioxidant properties of CBD/THC can minimize the plaque formation cycle associated with the progression of Alzheimer's disease. Research has shown that these antioxidant properties surpass the potency of either vitamin C or E. A study published in the Journal of Natural Products suggests that a combination of CBD and THC can fight off treatment-resistant bacteria such *Staphylococcus aureus* (MRSA) and tuberculosis.

---

6 Professor Raphael Mechoulam is the man who kick-started medical research in Israel and around the world. Since starting his research in 1960, he has been nominated for 25 academic awards.

Terpenes

The cannabis plant contains an amazing array of other components, including flavonoids, amino acids, fatty acids, and very importantly, terpenes.

Terpenes are volatile aromatic molecules that evaporate easily, but are easily noticeable through their smell. They give plants their unique fragrances.

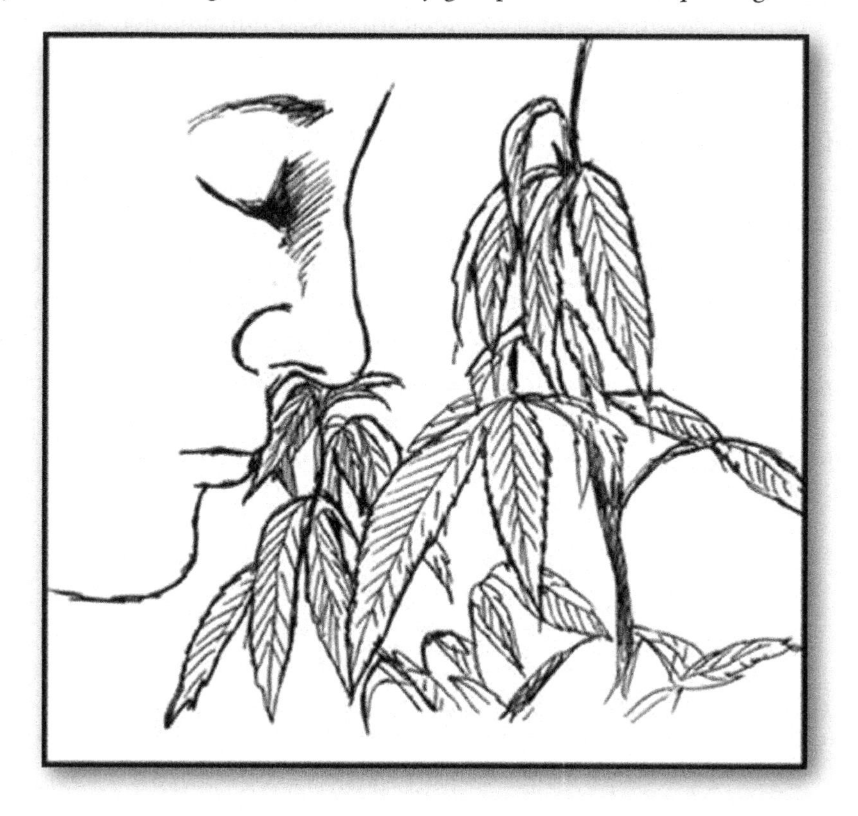

Basically, THC and the other cannabinoids themselves have no scent; the specific fragrance of a cannabis strain depends on which terpenes predominate. (Drug sniffing dogs are trained to smell terpenes, not THC.)

Terpenes are present naturally and abundantly in humans, plants and animals. So far, about 200 have been identified in cannabis. Only a few of these oily substances appear in sufficient strength to be significant, but a few of them show remarkable biological effects. In plants, they attract beneficial pollinating insects and repel predators and animal grazers; others prevent fungus.

But the influence of terpenes goes further. Some of them actually show anti-carcinogenic and anti-inflammatory effects. Supplementing the effect of the cannabinoids, some terpenes help to slow down cancer or help to prevent it in the first place. These effects are typically lacking in "CBD-only" products.

Terpenes have their own physiological effects, but they are most potent when they interact with other compounds in the plant. For instance, they can regulate how much THC reaches the brain, and even modify levels of dopamine and serotonin in the blood.

Limonene with its strong citrus fragrance is mood enhancing, strongly anti-fungal and known to work against cancer in a variety of ways. A review published in the *Journal of Nutrition* revealed that limonene helps prevent or delay breast, skin, liver, lung and stomach cancer in rodents.[7]

Terpenes can differ markedly from strain to strain. Patients who switch to another strain may not get the same beneficial effects if the terpene profile is considerably different.

---

7 Crowell, PL, Prevention and therapy of cancer by dietary monoterpens, *Journal of Nutrition* 129 (March 1999), 775S-778S.

Flavonoids

Cannabis also has over twenty flavonoids, which are chemicals common to most plant life. They are abundant in a variety of fruits and vegetables.

Flavonoids that are unique to cannabis are called cannaflavins. They are not just causing pleasant scents; like cannabinoids, they are pharmacologically active and have many beneficial biological effects. For a long time it was believed that these effects were due to their anti-oxidant properties. However, scientists at Oregon State University found this to be erroneous and stated that flavonoids "have little or no value in that role."[8]

For cancer patients, cannaflavins are beneficial because the human body identifies them as foreign substances and subsequently denatures or destroys them. This, in turn activates other chemicals, which also work to deactivate carcinogens. Thus, indirectly, flavonoids help to kill cancer cells and reduce tumor growth.

Cannaflavin A has been found to reduce inflammation by inhibiting the inflammatory molecule PGE-2, and it does this 30 times more effectively than aspirin.

Through complex biochemical mechanisms, flavonoids interact on many different sites in the body. Similar to CBD, they also help to lessen the psychoactive effect of THC.

8 Stauth, David, *Studies force new view on biology of flavonoids*, press release, Oregon State University, March 5, 2007.

Staying legal with the "Therapeutic Cannabis Recommendation"

Possession of cannabis is illegal in many countries as a result of the infamous agreement about *Indian hemp*, also known as hashish, at the International Opium Convention (1925). On the upside, more and more countries are decriminalizing the possession of cannabis. Others are permitting medical use of cannabis and are allowing medical users to grow their own personal supply.

In the US, the movement to end the shackles of cannabis prohibition continues to grow. Prohibition is crumbling under the pressure of science, facts and patient demand. Drug warriors and the DEA are losing the battle over medical marijuana because only diehard prohibitionists still believe their fabrications, and those numbers are shrinking.

As of January 2015, twenty-seven states and the District of Columbia have either legalized medical marijuana or decriminalized marijuana possession, or both. Despite the many years of Draconian anti-pot laws, more and more people are turning to cannabis for medical purposes.

Still, marijuana remains illegal under federal law. In the last decade, 6.5 million Americans have been arrested on marijuana charges, a greater number than the entire populations of Alaska, Delaware, the District of Columbia, Montana, North Dakota, South Dakota, Vermont and Wyoming combined. In 2012, state and local law enforcement arrested 749,825 people for marijuana violations. Since 2011, the Obama administration has shut down medical cannabis businesses throughout California on the grounds that the industry has spiraled out of control. In March 2014, the Drug Enforcement Administration raided several dispensaries in Los Angeles; a pot shop in Mendocino, closed by federal agents earlier last year, only recently reopened.

http://www.latimes.com/local/lanow/la-me-ln-marijuana-dispensary-raids-20140312,0,1390175.story - axzz2yJryJl5J.

Obama stated during a January 2014 *YouTube* interview that he suspects more states will look into legalization and promised a hands-off approach by federal agencies; yet things are still uncertain.

For that reason it is very important that cannabis users verify their countries' legal stance regarding cannabis breeding, and that they follow the rules and laws of the state in which they reside. This book is not written with the intent to encourage anyone to break the law.

California cannabis laws

In my home state California, PROPOSITION 215, the *Compassionate Use Act*, was enacted by the voters and took effect on Nov. 6, 1996 as *California Health & Safety Code 11362.5.*

SB420, a legislative statute, went into effect on January 1, 2004 as *California H&SC 11362.7-.83*. This statute broadens rights of medical patients by allowing them to form medical cultivation "collectives" or "cooperatives"; SB420 also establishes a voluntary state ID card system run through county health departments.

In October 2015 Governor Jerry Brown signed into law a legislative package of bills that would provide regulations for California's medical cannabis industry.

Under proposition 215, the following illnesses and diseases count as qualifying conditions:

- Arthritis
- Cachexia
- Cancer
- Chronic pain
- HIV or AIDS
- Epilepsy
- Migraine
- Multiple Sclerosis
- Any debilitating illness where the medical use of marijuana has been deemed appropriate and has been recommended by a physician.

What Proposition 215 and SB420 allow[9]

- Possession of up to eight ounces of dried cannabis.
- Cultivation of up to 12 plants, as long as 6 are mature at any given time. This pertains to the patients or the patients' primary caregiver.
- Cultivation should be indoors or in a locked greenhouse.
- Purchase and cultivation is allowed for personal use only.

To qualify as medical cannabis users, patients must obtain a California-licensed physician's "Recommendation" or "Approval" (NOT a prescription) to use marijuana.

A sample "Therapeutic Cannabis Recommendation" form is on the following page (they may vary slightly from doctor to doctor).

In California, the organization *Compassionate Health Options* has branch office locations throughout California. These offices have doctors on duty who are qualified to issue the "Therapeutic Cannabis Recommendations." For a separate fee, these offices also issue the optional "card."

Patients who are using cannabis without a doctor's recommendation may be breaking both state and federal law and leaving themselves open to harsh penalties. Even if they are using cannabis as a legitimate treatment for disease, they are still leaving themselves open to punishment if they do so without a California-licensed physician's recommendation.

Patients' officially designated caregivers are also eligible for so-called marijuana cards. A caregiver "is the individual, designated by a qualified patient or by a person with an identification card, who has consistently assumed responsibility for the housing, health, or safety of that patient or person. The caregiver must be 18 years of age or older (unless the primary caregiver is the parent of a minor child who is a qualified patient or a person with an identification card)." (http://norml.org/legal/item/california-medical-marijuana.)

9 Cannabis regulations often change from day to day. This book should not be taken as a source for legal or binding information on cannabis. Patients should always check federal, state and existing municipal laws and regulations.

Compassionate Health Options

Mental and Physical Wellness Counseling

Dr.

Therapeutic Cannabis Recommendation*

This certifies that ______________________________

born on ____________ (DOB), was examined in my office on 1/3/14 (Date Seen).

He/she was found to have a medical condition that in my professional opinion would benefit from the use of medical cannabis. I have discussed the potential risks and benefits of medical cannabis use as an appropriate therapeutic treatment pursuant to the Compassionate Use Act of 1996 (California Health & Safety Code 11362.5).

1) The patient understands and accepts the risks involved in using medical cannabis and will refrain from driving or engaging in any other potentially hazardous activity while impaired in any way.

2) The patient has been advised to use the least amount of cannabis needed. This medication should be used cautiously with alcohol or any other mind-altering substances.

3) It is understood that the patient will use discretion when using medical cannabis with respect to the rights of others.

The patient knows it is in his/her self-interest to seek further medical evaluation and treatment when appropriate. The patient authorizes Compassionate Health Options to discuss the contents of this letter for verification purposes only.

Diagnosis 327.81, 724.4, 724.2, 309.81,

This recommendation expires on 4/3/14

Signed ______________________

To **VERIFY** use this **ID #** ____________

www.GREEN215.com

1 877 PROP215 (877-776-7215)

A Medical Marijuana Identification Card—do I really need it?

It is true. In California patients only need the "Therapeutic Cannabis Recommendation." Nothing else. This protects them under PROPOSITION 215, the *Compassionate Use Act,* as well as under the *SB420* statute.

However, for greater peace of mind, many patients choose to also get a state-issued Medical Marijuana Identification Card. This is a wallet-size laminated card that easily fits into a billfold. The advantages are obvious:

- The MMIC identifies the cardholder as a person protected under the provisions of Prop 215 and SB420. It makes it simpler for law enforcement to identify the cardholder as a legal medical marijuana patient. For the patient, card carrying is less cumbersome than carrying around a laminated piece of paper like most doctors hand out.
- A medical marijuana card grants patients easy access to dispensaries.

Getting a regular Medical Marijuana Identification Card in California

In California, patients can get a regular Medical Marijuana Identification card through Medical Evaluation Centers, which are plentiful throughout the state. Patients can easily find Internet or phonebook listings for centers in their vicinity. All Medical Evaluation Centers have a doctor on their staff. Patients who do not have or know a cannabis-friendly doctor can get their "Therapeutic Cannabis Recommendation" right here.

California state-issued Medical Marijuana Identification Card

Alternately, patients may get a **state-issued** "Medical Marijuana Identification Card" (MMIC), although the process is somewhat more complicated. The government website for obtaining the MMIC is http://mmic.cdph.ca.gov/. As with the general MMIC, participation in the state card program is entirely voluntary. The California government website states:

> *"The California Department of Public Health's Medical Marijuana Program (MMP) was specifically established to create a State-authorized*

medical marijuana identification card (MMIC), along with a registry database for verification of qualified patients and their primary caregivers. The MMP Web-based registry allows law enforcement and the public to verify the validity of a qualified patient or primary caregiver's MMIC as authorization to possess, grow, transport, and/or use medical marijuana within California."

Warning! Beware of bogus clinics! Some unscrupulous doctors are charging for so-called "cultivation licenses." Allegedly, this permits cultivation of a larger number of plants than permitted by law. Under California law, there is no such thing as a "cultivation license," and no physician has the authority to prescribe plant numbers.

Other dishonorable clinics are run by doctors with invalid or suspended licenses, or under the proprietorship of non-physicians. This is against California law.

The healthiest way to consume medical cannabis

Back to my story. After choosing cannabis as my preferred medication, I had to decide how to administer it—smoking, vaporizing, topical application, using edibles, or suppositories. To ensure the most effective cancer killing approach, I tested various applications.

Smoking

Smoking still seems to be the most popular way of ingesting cannabis—even though it is not necessarily the healthiest approach.

The advantages of smoking are:

- The effect is felt almost immediately;
- It is easy to dose;
- For pain, it provided about 2 to 3 hours of relief;
- It is easy to use.

For a long time, there were conflicting opinions about smoking cannabis. Earlier government sponsored research alleged that marijuana smoke contains cancer-causing chemicals that could be potentially harmful to the lungs.

This view was finally disproven by a large study, which concluded that even heavy marijuana smoking does not lead to lung cancer.

Dr. Donald Tashkin of the University of California at Los Angeles carried out the study, and the *National Institute of Drug Abuse* funded it. It involved 1200 people in Los Angeles with lung, neck, or head cancer, and an additional

1040 people without cancer, matched by age, sex, and neighborhood. Tashkin presented the results in 2006 to a meeting of the American Thoracic Society in San Diego. According to Dr. Tashkin the results were very surprising. He stated:

> *"We hypothesized that there would be a positive association between marijuana use and lung cancer, and that the association would be more positive with heavier use. What we found instead was no association at all, and even a suggestion of some protective effect."*[10]

Dr. Tashkin speculated that perhaps the cannabinoids in marijuana themselves offset the carcinogens found in smoke. But despite the reassuring words by Dr. Tashkin, there are still significant disadvantages to smoking.

- Temperatures are reached through combustion. Combustion of cannabis releases toxic compounds and irritants. While inhaling them may not trigger cancer, it can still cause coughing and irritation of the respiratory tract.
- High combustion temperatures destroy most of the medicinal cannabis components without benefit to the patient.
- Constant use may be required throughout the day for chronic illnesses.
- It is dangerous to use outside of legal zones.

Because of the drawbacks, I decided to scratch smoking.

Vaporizing

Vaporizing cannabis is still one of the lesser-used techniques; probably, because it is more expensive than smoking. Yet, it has significant benefits, and there are many reasons why people are starting to switch:

- Vaporizers heat the cannabis without combustion. This causes the cannabinoids to be released into the air without any of the disadvantages

10 http://www.scientificamerican.com/article/large-study-finds-no-link/

of smoke. Precise temperature settings allow specific cannabinoids to be released and subsequently inhaled.

- Rather than burn plant material, vaporizers gently heat it to set temperatures. This releases the cannabinoids as a mild mist or vapor that can be inhaled. Because none of the cannabinoids are consumed by flame, patients receive nearly all of the medicinal benefits. With smoking, 88% of the combusted smoke gases contain non-cannabinoid elements. Conversely, vaporized gases consist of approximately 95% cannabinoids. The difference is HUGE.
- The lack of combustion protects inhalers entirely from the toxins that accompany smoking, such as carcinogenic tars and gases.
- Since the substance being inhaled is vapor, not smoke, there is no coughing associated with inhaling vaporized cannabis.
- Vapor is much purer than smoke and has a higher cannabinoid content. Some users claimed it produced a more clear-headed "high" due to the lack of smoke inhaled.
- Since vapor emits far less odor than smoke it is much more discreet.
- Pain relief tends to last longer than with smoking.
- Interestingly, many patients considered vaporizing as a more efficient way to use marijuana. Generally, smaller amounts of cannabis are required for vaporizing as compared to smoking or edibles.

A 2007 study at the San Francisco General Hospital concluded:

"Vaporization is a safe and effective cannabinoid delivery mode for patients who desire the rapid onset of action associated with inhalation while avoiding the respiratory risks of smoking, as they significantly reduce the intake of gaseous combustion toxins, including carbon monoxide."

VAPORIZING TEMPERATURES

Now this is a very important point. Cannabinoids are released at different temperatures. The recommended temperatures for vaporizing are:

- THC 284 to 320°F (140 to 160°C)
- CBD 320 to 356°F (160 to 180°C)
- CBN 365° F (185°C)
- CBC 428°F (220°C)

Warning! It is crucial not to heat the cannabis above 446°F (230°C); the substance starts to combust at this point and will release benzene and other harmful substances. This is outright dangerous!

Vaporizing is most economical

The fact that cannabinoids are activated at different temperatures makes vaporizing very economical.

Why? Let me explain.

For the full effect of their cancer killing potential, patients should ideally consume CBC, CBD, and THC strains. With a vaporizer this is very easily done because the individual strains are released at different temperatures.

Vaporizers do not burn the plant material, thus the load of the filling chamber can be re-heated several times at different temperatures until all the cannabinoids are completely dissolved.

This means that patients could start vaporizing for THC at the lowest temperature, and then re-vaporize the same plant material at the higher temperature for CBD. Later, they could re-vaporize one more time for CBN and last, at the highest temperature, for CBC. Because CBD, CBN and CBD have a higher release point than THC, they are not present in vapor produced at lower temperatures.

So by vaporizing cannabis with temperature controlled devices patients are using less plant but utilizing it better. Cannabis will last up to twice as long, which can make a big difference financially.

And as if this weren't enough, the remaining cannabis could yet be used in other cannabis preparations, such as edibles.

There you have it. For cancer patients vaporizing seems to be a very good option.

So, to start with, I decided to vaporize.

(Later on I decided to switch to cannabis oil, and I'll discuss that in later chapters. In fact, oil making became so important that I decided to devote several chapters to it.)

But right now I don't want to get ahead of myself, so let's get back to vaporizing.

Finding the best vaporizer

At this point, the next step for me was finding the most suitable vaporizer.

Vaporizers come in a variety of styles. The main difference is between stationary "table top" models and the portable or handheld styles. There are large numbers in each category advertised both on the Internet and in magazines.

Since I planned to use a vaporizer for a long time I wanted a quality product. I decided on a VOLCANO vaporizer from Storz & Bickel, a German company. Their main USA website is storz-bickel.com.

VOLCANO table top models come in either the digital or classic style. According to the description, the classic model probably works well, but since I wanted full control over the temperatures, and since I prefer ease of use, the VOLCANO DIGIT with the "Easy Valve set" was my personal choice.

The *VOLCANO DIGIT* Vaporizer

The "VOLCANO DIGIT" is very easy to operate. With the EASY VALVE SET, users do not even have to attach the balloon to the valve. Valve and balloon are already connected and the machine is ready to use. When the original EASY VALVE can no longer be used, it can simply be replaced with a new one. The EASY VALVE Starter Set comes with 5 EASY VALVE replacement balloons.

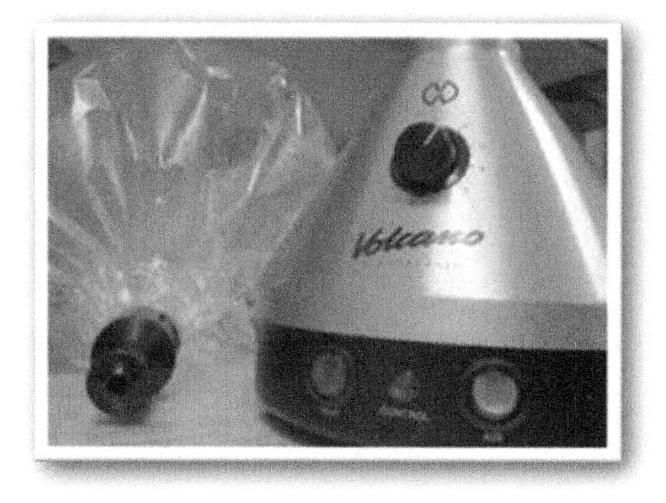

The simple design allows even novices to become experts in no time. According to testimonials, most users master the system in less than 10 minutes. But if there are questions, manufacturer support is easily available. The machine also comes with detailed instructions and a Quick Start Manual.

If several people want to use the same machine, additional "Valve Balloons with Mouthpieces" are available at a fair price.

VOLCANO vaporizers utilize patented technology to gently heat plant materials and fill a valve balloon with a fine mist or vapor that can be inhaled. The vapor produced is very pure and does not contain any dangerous combustion by-products like carbon monoxide. Chemical analysis (using VOLCANO vaporizers) showed that vapor contains fewer compounds overall, and the majority of toxins found in smoke were vastly decreased or absent.

Vaporization temperatures range between 104°F and 446°F (40°C and 230°C). The extra large, digital LED displays both the set and actual temperature. It usually takes between 30 seconds to 1 minute to fill a balloon. The automatic switch off after 30 minutes enhances security.

WARNING! Cheaper devices may heat inaccurately and may use plastic components in the vapor path. Heating plastic can release volatile toxins along with the vapor.

The VOLCANO creates only very mild odors compared to smoking. This means that non-smokers are not subject to any adverse effects when sharing rooms with other users.

The weight of the VOLCANO DIGIT is 4.0 lbs. (1.8 kg), and it comes with a three-year warranty.

Some vaporizers are very hard to clean. With the VOLCANO cleaning is effortless.

In quality and performance, the VOLCANO truly lives up to what one would expect of a German built machine. I honestly cannot find anything negative to say about it, except perhaps cost. Currently, prices rang from $539 to $669. Shipping via "UPS Next Day Air" from Oakland, California (for the US) is free on most orders. Admittedly, this seems expensive. But considering quality and performance it is hard, if not impossible, to find a better product. The VOLCANO DIGIT is truly the Rolls Royce of vaporizers.

The VOLCANO is often seen at cannabis events like the Cannabis Cup, where large, 5-foot long Volcano balloons are being displayed and passed around.

The PLENTY Vaporizer by Storz & Bickel

After about a month's use I liked the VOLCANO DIGIT so much that I decided to also order the portable PLENTY vaporizer. I like it because the PLENTY is a robust hand-held device, consisting of a Hot Air Generator and Vaporization Unit (the Filling Chamber with the cooling coil and a mouthpiece).

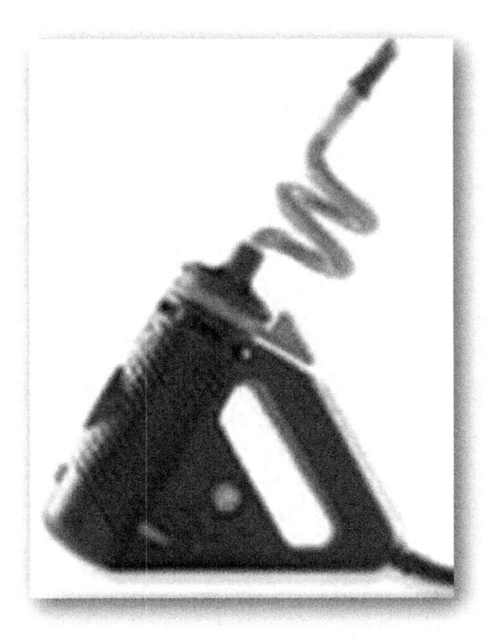

The PLENTY operates without any pumps or balloons. This makes the device very quiet and convenient to use. The heat exchanger is equipped with a double helix to ensure efficient air heating and high-yield vaporization.

The highly efficient stainless steel Cooling Coil ensures a pleasant aromatic experience.

With its weight of 1.5 lbs. (0.7 kg) it is easily portable. Although the PLENTY looks somewhat odd on the outside it functions incredibly well. It quickly became my favorite.

The temperature is adjustable through a rotating wheel on a scale from 1 to 7. The temperature range is from 266°F to 395°F (130°C to 202°C).

The highly effective stainless steel cooling coil ensures a pleasant aromatic experience, and the automatic switch-off ensures safety.

The PLENTY vaporizer costs $299. This includes the entire unit, and worldwide shipping is free.

Although, for myself, I had decided upon vaporizing, I want information for my readers to be as complete as possible. For that reason, I am going to describe two more methods of cannabis ingestion.

Ingesting "edibles"

Besides smoking or vaporizing, medical cannabis can be ingested in various kinds of foods and drinks, known as "edibles."

"Edibles" are food items made with cannabis, such as cookies, fudge, cupcakes and brownies. Aside from sweets, there are other items like pasta and sauces, or oils. "Canna butter" is regular butter that has been infused with fresh cannabis plant matter and can be used for home cooking.

Many patients prefer edibles because (a) the effect is longer lasting than other forms of medical marijuana and (b) there is no danger of the carcinogenic effects of smoking.

But aside from its advantages, edibles do have some drawbacks. The greatest problem seems to be with proper dosing.

Dr. Donald Abrams, M.D., Chief of Hematology and Oncology at San Francisco General Hospital and a cancer and integrative medicine specialist at the University of California/San Francisco, said that "it's much easier to regulate the onset and the effect of [medicinal marijuana] when you inhale it." He believes that many patients get into big trouble because they're not aware of the delayed onset of most edibles.[11]

Edibles are digested like food. This means that cannabinoids in food must move through the digestive process before being delivered into the bloodstream. They must then pass through the liver, which may convert THC into a more potent form and thus produce a stronger "high." Because of this lengthy and complex process, it is hard to assess dosage with edibles accurately. A marijuana brownie, for instance, may have a much stronger effect than three puffs from vaporizer or joint.

The effect of edibles is much slower to kick in, slower to wear off, and has an effect that many describe as *heavier* or *deeper* than from smoked marijuana. Generally, from edibles, patients don't feel the effect for 30 to 60 minutes, and if eaten after a meal, it may take nearly two hours for the full effect.

The "high" from edibles can last 4 to 8 hours while the effects from smoking can wear off in an hour or less.

---

11 Dr. Abrams has co-authored a textbook on the subject with Dr. Andrew Weil, titled *Integrative Oncology*. It is available on Amazon and Barnes and Noble for around $38.

To complicate the problem further, many edibles are baked by co-ops, collectives, or dispensaries; they are made with box mixes and whatever plant matter is available. Accordingly, the cannabis content can vary considerably from one batch to the next.

Conversely, smoked and vaporized cannabinoids enter the blood stream almost instantly. Since it is easy to stop inhaling once the desired effect is achieved these methods give patients much better control over dosing.

For accurate dosing, most doctors tend to recommend using a vaporizer over cannabis edibles.

Dr. Abrams has yet another concern—sugar. "Sugar does feed cancer!" he says, and unfortunately, most edibles contain sugar. "He says: "I personally believe that refined sugar and carbohydrates are not beneficial for individuals living with cancer because of their effect on insulin production and insulin-like growth factors, which promote inflammation and are also associated with cancer cell division."[12] Restricted access to glucose will compromise cancer cell growth and survival. Cancer cells must have glucose in order to live, and when they don't have glucose to nourish them, they die. Personally, I removed any kind of sugar, artificial sweeteners, or any insulin-enhancing products from my diet entirely. I will not even have them in the kitchen.

12 http://www.drweil.com/drw/u/ART03060/Treating-Cancer-With-Integrative-Medicine.html.

Rectal administration (suppositories)

Most people in the U.S. have a negative feeling towards rectal administration (suppositories). When I mention cannabis suppositories they typically have this look on their face: "You want me to put it WHERE?"

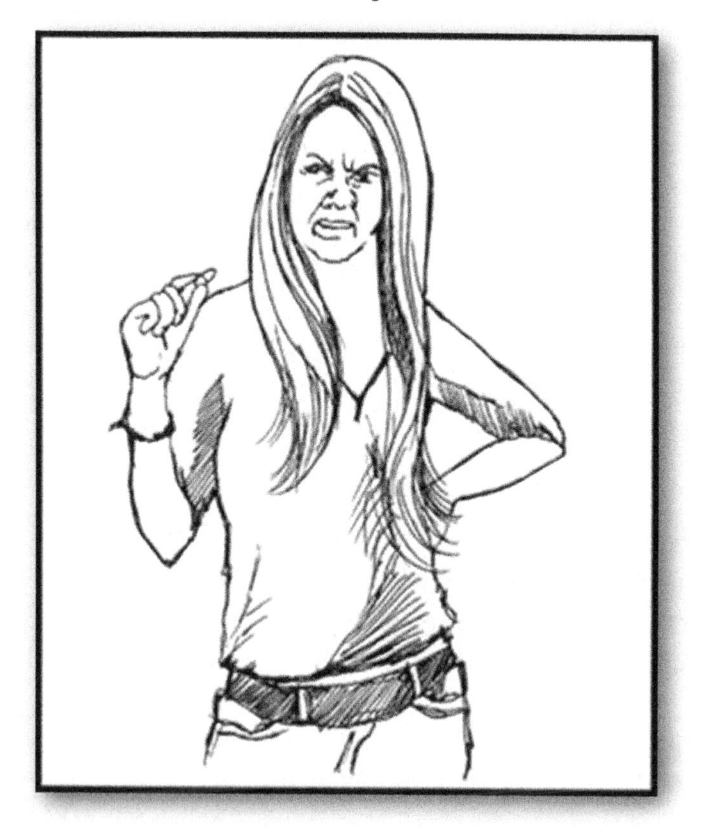

Yet there are many benefits associated with rectal administration. For instance:

- Medicine can be given when the oral route is impeded through nausea, mouth/throat difficulties, or because of gastrointestinal difficulties.
- Circumventing the gastrointestinal tract results in a higher level of active cannabis components to reach the blood in higher concentrations.

- Medicine can be applied "locally" in cases of tumors in the rectal cavity.
- Uptake into the blood stream is faster than with oral administration and leads to more consistent blood concentration of the cannabis components.

Rectal administration may enable individuals who have been unable to ingest cannabis via inhalation or ingestion to finally derive the therapeutic benefits of this amazing plant.

One colon cancer patient told me that she found this method very effective. "I want to put the medicine as close as possible to the cancer," she said.

It is important to realize that with suppositories patients can still feel the psychoactive effects of cannabis with high THC strains. In other words, they can still get "high."

I am ready to use cannabis–but where do I get it?

While cancer is a qualifying condition in all *legal* states, cancer patients make up only a small minority of medical cannabis users. In total, cancer patients appear to comprise less than 3% of total medical cannabis users in the US.

Having worked with cancer patients for about three years, I have found that one of the major reasons is the difficulty in obtaining the cannabis medicine. After obtaining a doctor's "Therapeutic Cannabis Recommendation," most patients have no idea where to go or what to do.

True, most communities (in *legal* states) have at least one or several dispensaries and most likely a number of marijuana delivery services. So there is no difficulty in getting cannabis. The problem is WHAT to get. Most of the marijuana products have such quirky or exotic names that for a medical patient they are more confusing than helpful.

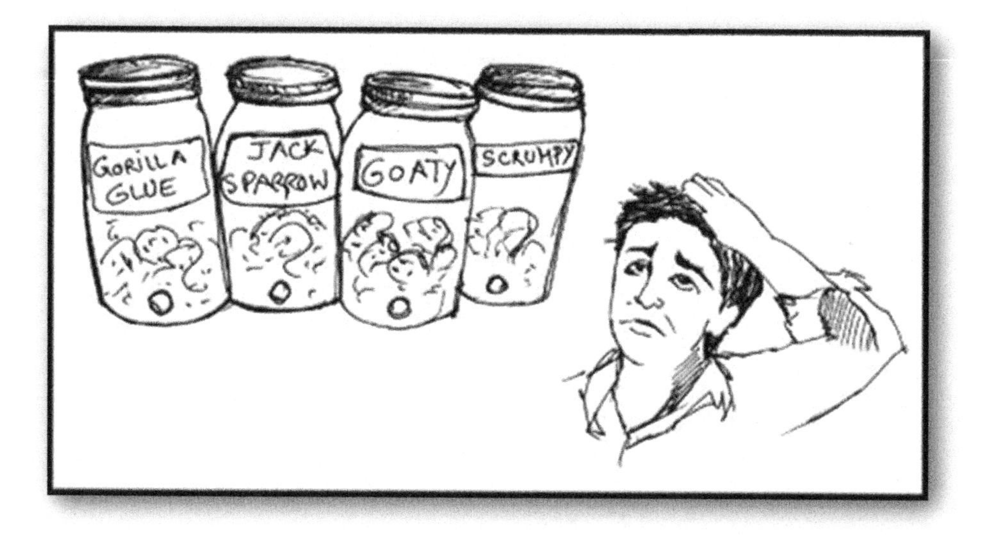

When you find yourself in such a situation, the following tips can help you:

Most dispensary strains are very high in THC. For cancer, you need both THC and CBD because both kill cancer in different ways. Therefore, your best choices would be indica/sativa hybrids, like

- Chem D
- Sour Diesel
- Bubba Kush
- Blue Dream or
- White Widow

Another therapeutically valuable strain is Harlequin, which is high in CBD.

I suggest that you ask a knowledgeable bud tender for strains grown from auto-flowering seeds. They invariably contain cannabis ruderalis, which is high in CBD.

All these strains can be used for vaporizing. But before you decide upon vaporizing, I suggest reading the next chapter about Cannabis Oil.

Cannabis oil—the most potent medicine

Even after I had started vaporizing I still was not fully convinced that I was taken the cannabis medicine in the most efficient manner. The more I researched the more I became convinced that cannabis oil was still more powerful.

After some experimenting I switched to oil entirely. (Today, I am only using oil made from my own strains. I will explain all this later on in the book.)

Cannabis oil is a thick, tar-like substance. Experience has shown that oil is more potent than vapor, smoke, or edibles because cannabis components are not only preserved throughout the extraction process; they are actually concentrated in the oil.

Preserving all cannabis components creates the famous "entourage effect," which was discovered by the Israeli researchers Ben-Shabat and Raphael Mechoulam and is being lauded by various researchers.

Unfortunately, cannabis oils available from various sources are not equal in quality or purity. Often oil is made from trim or parts of the plant that recreational growers would usually throw away.

Therefore, if at all possible, consider making your own cannabis oil. I recommend this to all cancer patients. (The picture shows a batch of freshly made cannabis oil—enough for five patients.)

If oil making is something you have never done, don't let that scare you—it is easier than you think. Just follow the instructions in the chapter "Step-by-step guide for making the oil." You will be well informed. I will guide you step by step without confusing you with complicated explanations. What you will learn will not be second-hand knowledge or guesswork. It will be practical information, based upon my own work, my own experiences—except I can save you the mistakes.

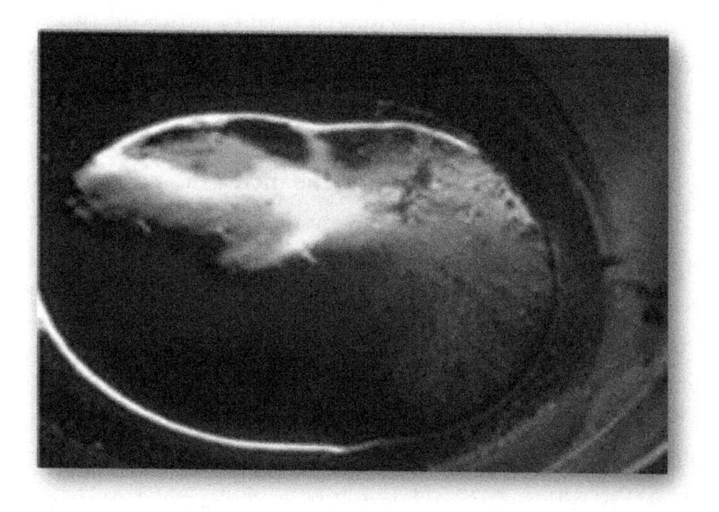

Cannabis oil can be vaporized, eaten straight, or put into easily ingested capsules. In each case, it retains the benefit of the whole plant components.

Cannabis oil is effective not only for cancer, but also for other serious ailments, like chronic pain, multiple sclerosis, fibromyalgia, arthritis, inflammation, Parkinson's disease, and a wide variety of age-related inflammatory and autoimmune diseases. Cannabis oil may also be useful in limiting neurological damage following a stroke or head injury. It is amazingly effective for insomnia.

Oil sold on the street should be avoided. More often than not, buyers will not know where the product originated. There is the risk that it could be infested with toxins, or cut with other products, such as vegetation or herbs. For a cancer patient, that could be outright dangerous. It is always more prudent to make your own oil or have someone you trust make it for you.

Also note that cannabis oil reacts negatively to light; it may lose its potency through extended exposure to light or heat. It is best stored in amber bottles, in a cool, dry and dark place.

Before delving seriously into oil-making specifics, a word of warning:

Beware of the industrial hemp oil hustlers

Since some promoters have been pushing "CBD oil only" products, the demand is skyrocketing; but true medicinal quality CBD oil (made from the genuine cannabis plant, not the industrial hemp plant) is notoriously difficult to find. This often leads desperate people to buy junk products with purported healing properties, but little or no science to back them up.

Unscrupulous people are exploiting the increasing popularity of CBD to produce oil from industrial hemp. They market their bogus product as "CBD-rich hemp oil" on the open market with very little fear of prosecution. They claim that it is the real thing because it contains CBD, or cannabidiol, which is one of the ingredients in marijuana that promotes healing. Except what they are using as the base of their oil is not exactly marijuana, but industrial hemp.

One "CBD-only" website states clearly: "Our oil is derived from the federally legal industrial hemp plant."

While technically, industrial hemp is from the same plant species that psychoactive marijuana originates from, it is from a different variety, or subspecies, and there are many significant deficiencies in the chemical compound.

The most serious shortcoming of industrial hemp oil is its lack of the "entourage effect." Israeli scientists Ben-Shabat and Raphael Mechoulamsay that "the basic idea of the entourage effect is that the various cannabinoids within the cannabis plant work together." Even though CBD oil hustlers oppose the idea, experiments have shown repeatedly that whole plant extractions are far more effective than CBD-only extractions.

Promoters typically insist that CBD-rich hemp oil is effective by itself, especially for children with severe epilepsy. This may be true, to some extent, but if your ailment is cancer, CBD from industrial hemp isn't going to be enough. Most serious illnesses require whole plant extracts, including THC.

Cancers, for instance, do need THC to shrink tumor cells and reduce the amount and severity of metastases.

Cristina Sanchez, a biologist at Complutense University in Madrid discovered that brain cancer cells died each time they were exposed to THC. Researchers found that THC induces apoptosis (self-killing of cancer cells) in leukemia cells. Peer-reviewed studies in several countries showed that THC is effective not only for cancer-symptom management (nausea, pain, loss of appetite, fatigue), it also exerts a direct antitumor effect.

The reason for the low THC content in industrial hemp is that most THC is formed in resin glands on the buds and flowers of the female cannabis plant. Industrial hemp is not cultivated for producing buds but rather for the long stems to be used for fiber. It therefore lacks the primary component to form the THC.

The greatest danger, however, lies in the fact that the so-called legal "CBD-rich hemp oils" are often derived from industrial hemp byproducts, usually imported as "refined sludge" from China, but also from Eastern Europe. Since hemp is a "bio-accumulator"—meaning the plant naturally draws toxins from the soil—some of the industrial hemp is grown for bio-remediation, meaning that the plant is used to leach heavy metals out of poisoned soil. Many of these contaminants are then retained in the hemp slush or paste and subsequently, in the oil.

A very disturbing Facebook post (since removed) from a former head of a "CBD-only" manufacturing plant was published on November 20, 2013:

> *I'm tired of so called CBD companies claiming that what they provide is medicine. Anyone using a CBD from hemp product please be aware of what you're actually getting is not what you think. These formulations start with a crude and dirty hemp paste (contaminated with microbial life! I have seen this and these organisms decompose the paste. The paste perhaps even contains residual solvent and other toxins as the extraction is done in China) made in a process that actually renders it unfit for human consumption.*
>
> *What these bogus companies are doing is criminal and dangerous. In fact [name of the oil] is literally just this hemp paste diluted in hemp seed oil. No refinement at all!!! And what [another company name] is offering is beyond disturbing. I cannot keep quiet any more. And since I formulated most of these products, I feel responsible for spreading the truth. I left [the company] for ethical reasons but it is not enough to just walk away. These frauds need to be exposed for what they are...*

It's against federal law to use hemp leaves and flowers to make drug products. Hemp oil entrepreneurs attempt to sidestep this legal hurdle by dubiously claiming they extract CBD only from hemp stalks before importing it to the United States, a grey area activity at best.

"CBD-rich hemp oils" are being sold to unsuspecting people for staggering amounts. A current advertisement quotes $549 per tube or six tubes for $3,294. Cannabis insiders have known about the CBD con game for a long time. But the mothers and fathers, the housewives, the newcomers, and especially many cancer patients and the elderly don't know about this. All they know is that someone is sick, and there may be a glimmer of hope with cannabis. In their time of need, unprincipled types rip off these vulnerable people and con them out of their hard earned cash.

"The atmosphere around marijuana in America right now is a perfect storm for fraud, corruption, and deception," wrote East Bay-based marijuana activist Mickey Martin in a blog post earlier last year.

Oil, oil, oil–I am totally confused

At this point, all this talk about the different kinds of oil may seem a confusing. Let's take a closer look.

Before we even start, let's understand that all these oils get their names from the plants from which they are extracted.

Cannabis oil is extracted from the genuine cannabis plant, which is grown for its potent, resinous glands. The cannabis plant contains numerous cannabinoids, foremost among them the psychoactive CBD and THC. It is from this plant species that true medical cannabis oil is derived.

Typically, cannabis oil is a whole plant extraction, which includes THC, CBD, and other cannabinoids and additionally more than 400 trace compounds. These other compounds interact synergistically to create an "entourage effect" that can magnify the therapeutic benefits of the individual components

Hemp seed oil is extracted from food-grade hemp plants, which are grown specifically for their seeds. The seeds are made into oil as well as into various food products, such as flour, pasta, cereal, etc. Shelled hemp seeds are sold as delicious snacks in various varieties. The important point is that hemp seed oil and hemp seed food products are made only from the seeds.

Hemp oil is usually extracted from the industrial hemp plant. The hemp plant is foremost grown for fiber and is used to produce thousands of items such as rope, paper, clothing, and even bio fuel.

The industrial hemp plant contains a minuscule amount of THC (less than 0.3%), and a higher concentration of CBD. Because of state and federal laws allowing sale of oil that is low in THC and high in CBD, unscrupulous people are marketing "CBD-rich Oil" or "Hemp Oil" made from industrial hemp for medicinal purposes. The unsuspecting public does not know that this oil is, in reality, a byproduct of large-scale hemp stalk and fiber processing facilities in Asia and Europe. More often than not, it is imported as "refined sludge" and may be contaminated (as has been explained in the previous chapter).

Unwary buyers may think that they are buying medicinal CBD oil without realizing that 100 milligrams of industrial hemp-derived CBD oil is not equivalent to 100 milligrams of a CBD-rich whole plant cannabis extract.

Genuine cannabis oil can only be sold with a doctor's therapeutical recommendation (in "legal" states). If Hemp Oils or CBD-rich Oils are sold freely without restrictions, they are most likely derived from industrial hemp. With Hemp Oil and especially CBD-only oils it is strongly recommended that BUYERS BEWARE!

Making cannabis oil—it's easier than you think

If you are an absolute beginner—making oil is easier than you think. But please read this section very carefully. Before you start making oil you really should know this.

And even if you are an experienced oil maker, you may want to review this section. Chances are you will see at least a few things you've forgotten that will come in handy now that you've been reminded of them.

And don't forget that making cannabis oil still falls under a gray area of marijuana possession. Follow the legal guidelines for making the oil; be sure that you can prove it is for medical uses and not for illegal substance abuse or distribution.

Cannabis oil extraction—which solvent is best?

Cannabis oil is made by extracting therapeutic cannabis compounds with a solvent. Next, the solvent is evaporated, leaving behind a tar-like substance resembling oil.

Almost all oil makers are essentially using the same extraction process, except that they use different kinds of solvents.

Rick Simpson advocated the use of naphtha or petroleum ether. Many experts believe that these solvents create unnecessary hazards for patients. Both are mixtures of benzene, hexane, etc., which are considered carcinogenic. Moreover, naphtha-based cannabis oil contains a lower concentration of terpenes and a much higher percentage of decarboxylated tetrahydrocannabinol (THC) compared to oil made with other extracts.[13]

---

13 Decarboxylation is a chemical (heating) process that converts THCa into THC, the compound that causes the psychoactive effects.

Alternative methods are ethanol, food grade alcohol, olive oil, coconut oil, etc. Lab studies at the University of Siena (Italy) concluded that "ethanol and olive oil were determined to be the most effective, largely because of their ability to produce an extract with a high terpene content. Then too, both substances are safe for consumption." For my SHORAK oil production I use only food grade alcohol as solvent. (You will learn about SHORAK oils in great detail later on in the book.)

THINGS YOU WILL NEED FOR MAKING OIL

- Plant material (about 1 pound or 448 grams[14])

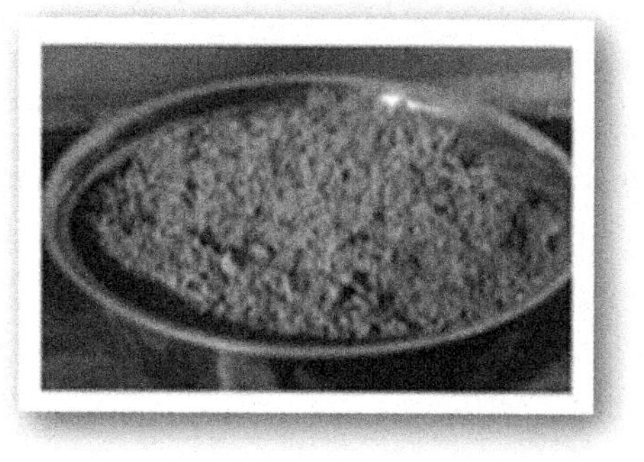

- Coffee filters (available for 10-gallon urn, 23"x9") at www.Amazon.com

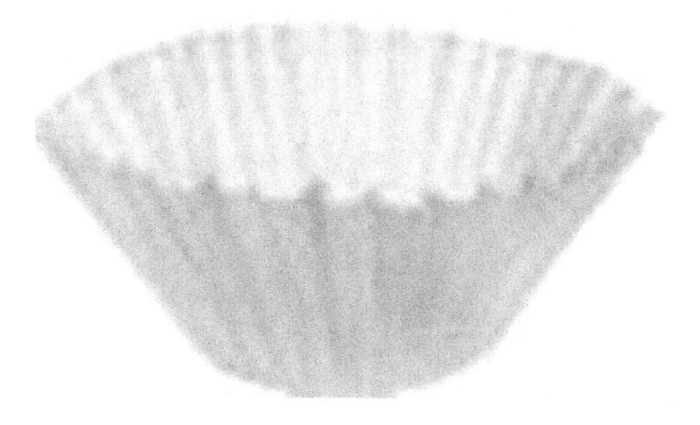

14 Using the standards used in the cannabis industry, an ounce is 28 grams, a quarter pound 112 grams and four of those add up to 448 grams, which is actually a little short of a pound—but it's the way the cannabis industry figures.

- 91% (or higher) Isopropyl rubbing alcohol
- Electric rice cooker or Induction cook top

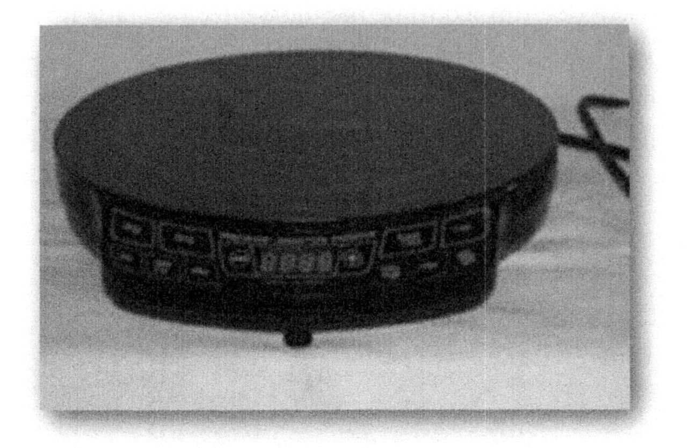

- High heat gloves or oven mitts
- Containers for holding oil (unless you put them into syringes right away)
- Large stainless steel bowls
- Non-latex safety gloves
- Oral dispensing syringes

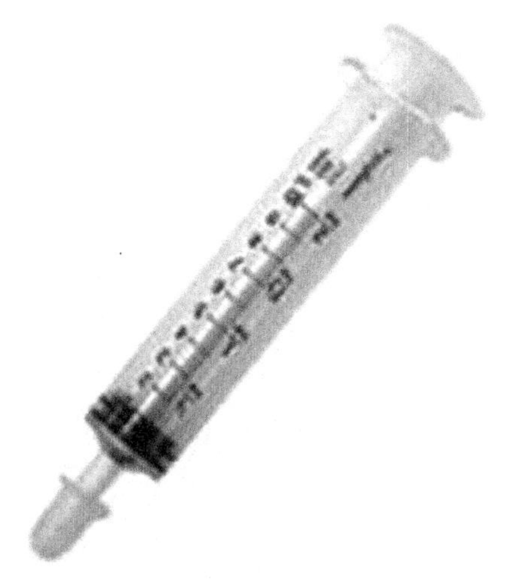

(*Kendall Monoject Oral Medication Syringes--Type - Clear - Capacity - 10ml/ 2 tsp.* — available from www.Amazon.com)

- Respirator mask (to be worn while evaporating alcohol)
- Stainless steel mesh strainer (select according to amount of material to be strained)
- Stainless steel mixing spoons with long handle
- Fire extinguisher at the place where you evaporate the alcohol

Step-by-step guide for making cannabis oil

METHOD ONE: Freezing extraction

1. Place ground up cannabis plant material in freezer (in plastic bag) overnight.
   - Place alcohol in freezer overnight
   - Use at least 32 oz. per ounce of cannabis, because the alcohol gets quickly saturated.
   - Get a stainless steel pot large enough to hold everything according to how much plant material you want to use.
   - Put cannabis in pot.

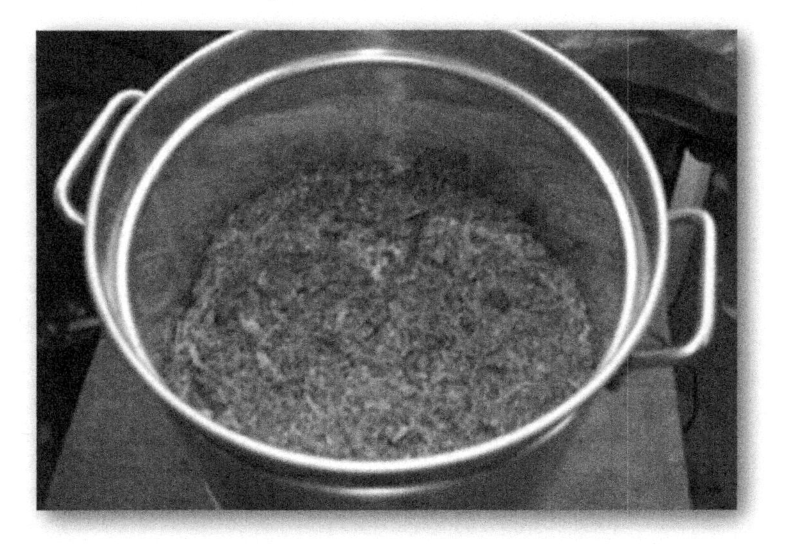

   - Pour frozen alcohol over it, stir it, make sure cannabis is well crushed up (use a sterile stirring rod or spoon).

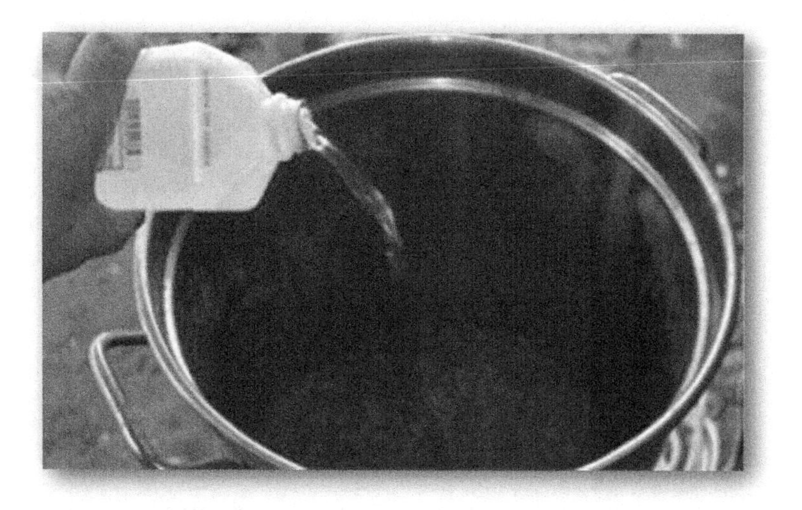

- Place pot with cannabis and alcohol in refrigerator for four hours and stir every thirty minutes.
- Take mesh strainer and put coffee filter in it (or use piece of cloth, like from a t-shirt, or cheese cloth, or something like that).

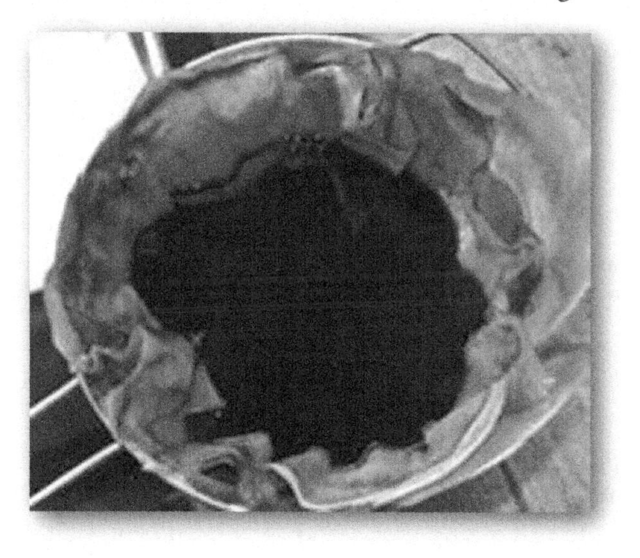

- Pour frozen mixture (alcohol and cannabis) through it, straining out the cannabis.
- Dump cannabis plant material back in pot.

- Pour a little more frozen alcohol over it and stir it, to make sure to get out any remaining alcohol. That could be as much as 20%.
- Strain it again.
- Take clean strained alcohol/cannabis and put it in clean stainless pot (or better a large stainless steel bowl).

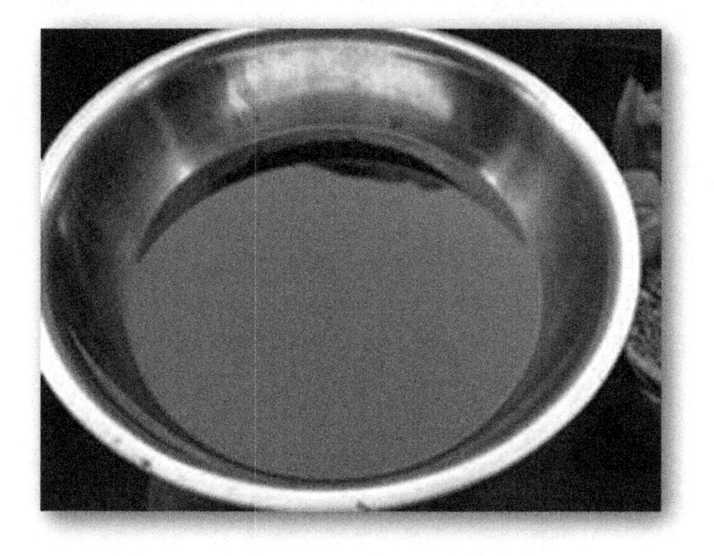

Extremely important! Do this outside only. Ensure that a fire extinguisher is nearby to quickly extinguish flames. Do not use water since this is an oil-based process. (Use baking soda or flame retardant powder instead).

- No cigarette smoking in the immediate area!
- Use hotplate (preferably Precision Induction cook top—it is the safest one for evaporating away the alcohol.)
- Place bowl on hotplate with filtered alcohol/oil mixture.
- Turn hotplate to about 180 degrees.
- Slowly evaporate away the alcohol (could take a couple of hours).
- As you start to get near bottom, turn temperature down slowly to 175°.
- Eventually the mixture will get really thick with little bubbles in it.

- The 91% (or higher) alcohol is being used because it contains a small amount of water. The water guarantees you that all of the alcohol will be long gone before the water ever is. This way you can be sure to end up with alcohol-free oil. If you are using 99% alcohol, add a few drops of water.
- When the bubbling in the oil stops, the oil is ready for consumption.

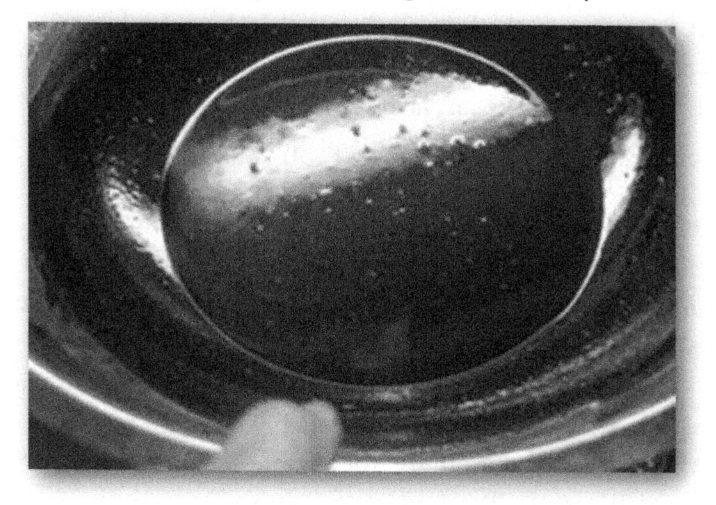

If the final product tastes like a dead skunk soaked in Diesel it is perfect. If you think I am kidding, wait until you taste it.

With METHOD ONE, you will get a higher THC content, but you will not get as much oil as with METHOD TWO.

METHODTWO: Hot extraction
Extremely important! Do this outside only.

1. Take stainless steel pot, place crushed up cannabis in the pot.
2. Pour alcohol over cannabis.
3. Turn cooktop to 190 degrees (if you are using Induction cook top)
   (If you are using a rice cooker, have it just hot enough where the alcohol mixture boils without burning the mixture. Higher priced rice cookers usually have a thermostat to keep rice from burning.)

4. Boil the alcohol with the cannabis for at least two hours.
5. Filter like before (under Method ONE, #6 and #7).
6. Evaporate alcohol away like in Method ONE (#16).

Be sure to use sufficient solvent; alcohol can hold only so much oil before it becomes over-saturated.

Both extraction methods work; except that the second one is more traditional. I admit I am somewhat old school when it comes to making oil. That's why METHOD TWO is my favorite. And I like it that with METHOD TWO I am getting more oil out of the plant material.

How much oil should I make?

For a cancer cure, most experts recommend 60 grams of cannabis oil to be taken within 90 days. After working with cancer patients for nearly three years, I developed a marvelously effective protocol including an additional 26 grams of oil for pre-treatment and post-treatment procedures. For 86 grams of oil you would need 448 grams of plant material.

(For detailed information see the chapter: "The complete SHORAK Cannabis Oil Treatment Plan for Cancer" in this book.)

Dosage for taking cannabis oil for cancer

After my own healing I started sharing oil with friends and patients in the cancer support group.

From a patient:
Do please know that the oil is simply fantastic; the results around the cancer are amazing. It is all stabilized, contained and seems to be neutralized. That is a blessing and relief. Regards, Matt

Most patients with whom I shared the oil were appreciative, but from the beginning, there was this giant stumbling block. It was nearly impossible to get patients to take the correct dose at appropriate times.

Because cannabis oil is so concentrated, it is prudent to start with a very small dose, about the size of half a grain of dry rice. Even if there is initially no obvious effect, patients can be assured that the oil is working.

However, in spite of detailed instructions from me, patients kept taking more than the suggested dose. They seemed to think, "If a little oil is so good, more would be even better."

But with cannabis this is not true. Cannabis oil works on microscopic levels, and taking high doses can actually be counter-productive. **Recent studies have shown that consistently high doses of cannabis cause the brain to reduce the density of cannabis receptors in the body, apparently in response to these high doses**. The body reduces the number of receptors in order to re-establish balance to the endocannabinoid system.

Here is a simple general rule: "Use the smallest possible dose required for the medical need, and complete the treatment course in the shortest possible time at that dose in order to avoid the chance of the patient developing overdosing tolerance issues."

Overdosing

This is a short section because lethal overdosing with cannabis is most unlikely.

It is true that small doses are recommended, but even if taken in larger amounts, cannabis is a remarkably safe drug. Unlike alcohol, opiates, and many pharmaceutical medicines, cannabis is not known to cause fatal overdoses. The estimated lethal dosage adds up to smoking 1,500 pounds in about 15 minutes. Yet, even if you took in such as strong dose you would still survive because there are no cannabinoid receptors in the brain stem, the part of the brain that controls vital functions such as breathing and heartbeat. Fact is, even strong doses of cannabis do not endanger life.

The effects of over-consuming cannabis will wear off without detrimental long-term effect; however, the immediate effect tends to be unpleasant for some patients.

Francis Young, administrative judge of the DEA, in his 1988 recommendation for legalizing marijuana, wrote: "Marijuana in its natural form, is one of the safest therapeutically active substances known to mankind."

Bi-phasic effect of CBD

Another reason for watching dosing carefully is that the phytocannabinoid CBD (plant CBD) has a biphasic effect. This means that small and high doses cause opposite reactions. An easy example for this is alcohol. Up to a blood level of 0.5% alcohol lifts mood and stimulate; drinkers become less constrained, and more cheerful, and happy. However, once drinkers exceed the 0.5% threshold the effects is the opposite, drinkers start feeling "down," or depressed. It is the same way with CBD, where small doses and high doses have opposite effects.

Why can't I take the oil in one single dose?

Over and over patients keep asking why they cannot not simply take the daily amount of cannabis oil in one single dose, preferably in the evening.

The reason is that a single dose is not nearly as effective.

Healing with cannabinoids is most successful if constant pressure is kept on the cancer. A single dose lasts about 6 hours, depending on potency. Dosing only once a day gives the cancer an 18-hour period where it is not being treated fully and one 6-hour period where the cancer has cannabinoid pressure via your daily dose.

Dividing the amount to be taken into 4 individual doses keeps continuing pressure on the cancer.[15]

The important role of Omega-3's

My treatment protocol includes hempseed oil in the starter dose and in the mixture for the pre-treatment and post-treatment phases. This is very important.

Here is why.

Hemp seed oil (oil made from the hemp **seed**, not cannabis oil made from the plant and—heaven forbid!—not oil made from industrial hemp) contains all the essential amino acids necessary for human life. It is rich in iron and vitamin E. It also provides trace minerals including calcium, iron, magnesium, manganese, potassium, phosphorus, sulfur and zinc. It delivers chlorophyll and carotene, a precursor to vitamin A, as well.

15 See the chapter "The Complete SHORAK Cannabis Oil Treatment Plan for Cancer."

Most importantly, hemp seed oil has the most perfectly balanced spectrum of omega-6 and omega-3 essential fatty acids (E.F.A.'s)

Essential Fatty Acids are crucial for health and vitality. But our bodies cannot make them, so they must be included in the diet on a regular basis. It is estimated that more than 90% of Americans take in too little of the important EFA Omega-3. Chances are that you might be deficient in Omega-3 yourself.

This is even more crucial for medicinal cannabis users. Omega-3 could make the difference between health and sickness!

Why?

Because humans need Omega-3 for properly functioning CB1 receptors. With failing or improperly functioning CB1 receptors, cannabis is less efficient at healing!

Omega-3 fatty acids are among the building blocks, which the body uses to make, maintain, and repair its own endocannabinoids. Lacking sufficient Omega-3, CB1 receptors get broken or "uncoupled." Impaired CB1 receptors have been connected to Huntington's disease, Alzheimer's, premature birthing, intestinal tumors, Parkinson's, inflammation-related ailments, risk of heart failure, atherosclerosis, rheumatoid arthritis symptoms, childhood development problems and certain cancers. Other symptoms are growth retardation, impairment of vision and learning ability, poor coordination, tingling in arms and legs, as well as mood swings and behavioral changes. Some researchers claim that Omega-3 acids are anti-aging. Others assert that they boost brain health and help to prevent or lessen depression.

Granny Storm-Crow, an international cannabis activist, wrote :

> *"The US diet sucks big time and we are fat, undernourished, and crazy because of it. We get WAY too much Omega 6 and not enough Omega 3. Not getting enough Omega 3 can make you crazy because without it, the CB1 cannabinoid receptors in your brain aren't made right- a chunk that is supposed to be attached, isn't! Broken receptors give you "impaired emotional behavior". So we think it's the low Omega 3 diet is making the US totally nuts!"*

But I have good news for you.

All this is can be turned around. Just two tablespoons of hempseed oil per day can bring your Essential Fatty Acids (E.F.A.'s) into balance. Cannabis has the ability to cause new cell growth in the brain and, with sufficient Omega-3, in only three to four weeks defective CB1 receptors will be replaced with new healthy ones. It takes about a month for effects to show up medically.

> *Hemp seeds contain the most balanced and richest natural single source of essential oils for human consumption. The E.F.A.'s (essential fatty acids) not only help to restore wasting bodies, but also improve damaged immune systems. (Eidlman, M.D., Hamilton, Ed.D., Ph. D., 1992*

Hemp seed oil is easily available in health food stores.. My preferred brand is Nutiva Organic Hemp oil. (A 24-ounce bottle sells for $20.68 at www.Amazon.com.).

SHORAK Cannabis Treatment Protocol

(SHORAK is the brand name for my own cannabis strains and seeds.)

How the SHORAK Protocol differs from other treatment plans

The general consensus is that cancer patients require a total of 60 grams of cannabis oil for treatment. This amount is to be ingested over a period of 90 days.

However, experience has shown that many new patients have difficulties getting used to ingesting cannabis. Things get even more problematic when (as some dispensaries recommend) THC and CBD are taken separately. This tends to produce undesirable side effects from THC, like disorientation, drowsiness, dizziness, accelerated heart rate, etc.

Because of these difficulties I made significant changes to my own SHORAK oil treatment plan.

1. I added a "STARTER DOSE," consisting of 1 gram of cannabis and 6 grams of hempseed oil.
2. I added two 10-gram syringes with milder, but still powerful cancer-killing strains to ease patients into the full treatment cycle. (The ratio is 5 grams of cannabis to 5 grams of hempseed oil.)
3. I added another three 10-gram syringes with the same mild oil for post therapy maintenance.

These items are provided in addition to the 60 grams of oil for the actual therapy cycle. To my knowledge, they are not included with any other program on the market.

The difference, however, is huge. The modified protocol has effectively eliminated nearly all starting difficulties. The patients I support are now beginning their full treatment program without difficulties.

1. Beginning phase

Starter dose (cannabis plus hempseed oil)

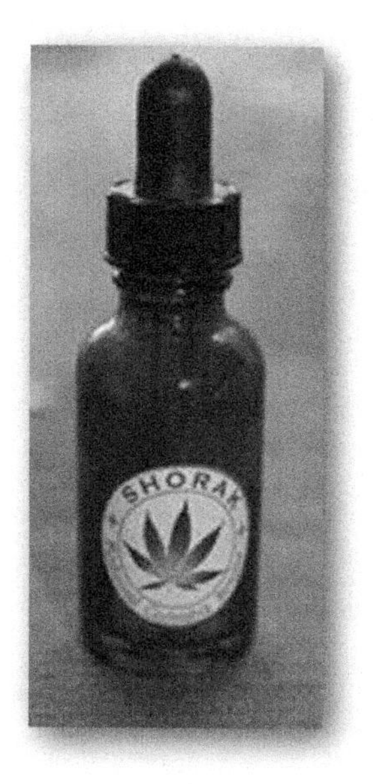

Take the 7 grams of cannabis/hempseed oil within 7 days at 1 gram per day.

This amounts to about 25 drops per day.

Divide this into 5 individual dosages of 5 grams; take throughout the day.

- Using this method allows the body to build up its tolerance slowly.
- Low initial doses enable the body to "wake up" the body's CB receptors.
- The addition of hemp seed oil is beneficial since it contains the richest and most balanced natural single source of essential oils for human consumption. The E.F.A.'s not only help to restore wasting bodies, but also improve damaged immune systems.

2. Pre-treatment phase

MILD CANNABIS OIL(2 SYRINGES)

Start the Pre-treatment phase with the two syringes marked "M"(mild). This is a milder, but very effective strain that will help you to transition easily into taking cannabis full strength.

Take 0.66 grams (about 16 drops) per day. Take in 4 individual doses of 4 drops.

Take until both syringes are finished.

Keep all oils refrigerated.

3. Full treatment phase

FULL STRENGTH CANNABIS OIL (6 SYRINGES)

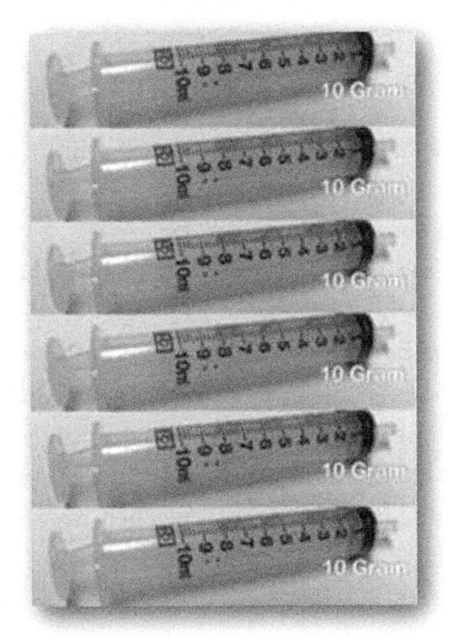

This is full-strength cannabis oil.

Take the full-strength oil (6 syringes at 10 gram each) within 90 days.

This amounts to .66 grams (16 drops) per day. Take the oil in 4 individual doses of 4 drops. This will amount to 59.4 grams in 90 days.

Keep refrigerated.

For serious cancer cases, try to speed up the process so that you are taking a minimum of 1 gram of oil per day as quickly as possible. This is very important. One gram equals about 25 drops of oil.

We like for people to stay within their comfort zone, but truth is, if you are very ill, the faster you can ingest the oil, the better your chances for surviving. (Remember, this is only for very sick patients.)

Important! If you find it difficult to take the oil "straight," you can alternately put it into gelatin capsules

("Empty Gelatin Capsules 0 Size" — available at www.Amazon.com.)

4. Post-treatment phase

MILD CANNABIS OIL (3 SYRINGES)

After finishing the treatment phase, it has been proven beneficial when patients stay on a maintenance dose to keep the cancer at bay.

Take about 5 drops of the mild cannabis oil per day until the three syringes have been finished.

The maintenance dose will also help to revitalize your body and lessen the damage that is often done through chemotherapy and radiation.

After very serious or multiple cancers, patients may choose to stay on the maintenance dose for a much longer time.

Important words about dosing

One of the hardest facts to impress on patients is to take exactly the suggested dose. Most patients are inclined to take too much oil.

On the other hand, there are a few who feel they have to "flood" the body. We actually had a caretaker who tried to give her husband half a syringe of oil every day.

Cannabis oil works on microscopic levels. While the recommended dose has been proven to be maximally effective, overdosing is counter-productive. Recent studies have shown that consistently very high doses of cannabis cause the brain to reduce the density of cannabis receptors in the body, apparently in response to these high doses. The body reduces the number of receptors in order to re-establish balance to the endocannabinoid system.

The suggested doses have proven to be the most effective ones for cancer treatment; so it is prudent to follow instructions carefully.

Bonus: coconut-infused cannabis oil

Growing evidence has shown that *Organic Virgin Coconut Oil* provides extraordinarily powerful anti-inflammatory, anti-biotic, anti-viral, anti-fungal, and immune-boosting properties.

For patients with neuropathy or especially painful cancers, we include a container of coconut infused cannabis. The ointment contains high quality cannabis oil infused into Organic Virgin Coconut oil.

The ointment can be applied topically or ingested. For topical use, take the needed amount of oil out of the container and let it warm to room temperature for easier spreading.

Because we recognize that many users are sensitive to fragrances we offer only an unscented version.

Commitment-doing your part

Cannabis is an amazingly powerful remedy, and cannabis oil has nearly miraculous healing properties. Still, as a cannabis patient, you have to be fully committed to do your part, and you have to be determined to follow through. A hit and miss program will not work. If you start, you can let nothing and no one interfere. If the schedule calls for 4 doses per day, you must take all four of them at the specified time and at the specified dose. Excuses like, "I have to run an errand," or "I have to drive somewhere and cannot take the oil" or "I can feel the oil and I don't like that feeling," are not acceptable. Momentary enthusiasm is of no value. If you want—REALLY want—to cure yourself, all you have to do is start the program and stick to it.

Important message

We do not sell oil. We help cancer patients who want to use the oil as cancer treatment, and who do not have the opportunity or the necessary knowledge to make it themselves. This is strictly a labor of love by a former cancer patient, who cured himself with cannabis oil, and who is giving his time and knowledge to help other cancer patients.

At a cannabis dispensary you would have to pay between $7,200 to $9,600 for the same amount of oil made out of dispensary pot, which most likely would only be single strain oil. SHORAK oils contains 2 to 20 (or possibly more) different medicinal strains.

We appreciate and depend upon donations to cover the manufacturing cost to keep this program going.

SHORAK cannabis oils ingredients

Not all cannabis oils are alike. A European friend just recently sent this message: "Unfortunately, we aren't seeing the miracles from the Cannabis I can get in Europe as the people at your end are seeing with SHORAK oil. It is so sad that these people are taking the stuff but it isn't really curing them. It seems to give them some relief but I don't see it regressing the tumors in the way you do."

While our specially prepared SHORAK cannabis oil is somewhat similar to the well-known RSO (Rick Simpson Oil), it differs greatly in important ways:

- SHORAK oil is made only from organically grown and carefully bred and selected cannabis strains with high therapeutic value, including the finest THC and CBD-rich strains. This careful selection process ensures the largest spectrum of therapeutically active cannabinoids.

- In contrast, RSO oil is often made from whatever pot is available, including from brick weed, which may or may not include dangerous amounts of pesticides, additives or mold.
- For SHORAK oil extraction we use exclusively 91% or higher Isopropyl Alcohol which is safe for consumption.
- Rick Simpson, on the other hand, advocated the use of Naphta as a solvent. Naphta, is a dangerous combustible petroleum product, which can be harmful to patients; it is illegal in California.
- The SHORAK extraction method with 91% or higher Isopropyl Alcohol produces an extract with a much higher medicinally valuable terpene content.
- The RSO extraction method with Naphta has been proven to result in a much lower concentration of terpenes.

Both SHORAK oil and the coconut infused cannabis oil ointments are hand-made. They contain no alcohol, no artificial fragrances, and no petroleum products.

We absolutely do NOT use industrial hemp or cannabis grown by unknown growers.

The "Therapeutic Cannabis Recommendation"

We can only help patients with a legal "Therapeutic Cannabis Recommendation" from a California-licensed medical doctor. Also, during Cannabis treatment, patients should be monitored and supervised by medical professionals at all times.

Caution: Medicinal Cannabis oil may be strong; therefore, it is advisable to not operate machinery or drive.

Cannabis oil should be stored in a cool, dry place, preferably refrigerated.

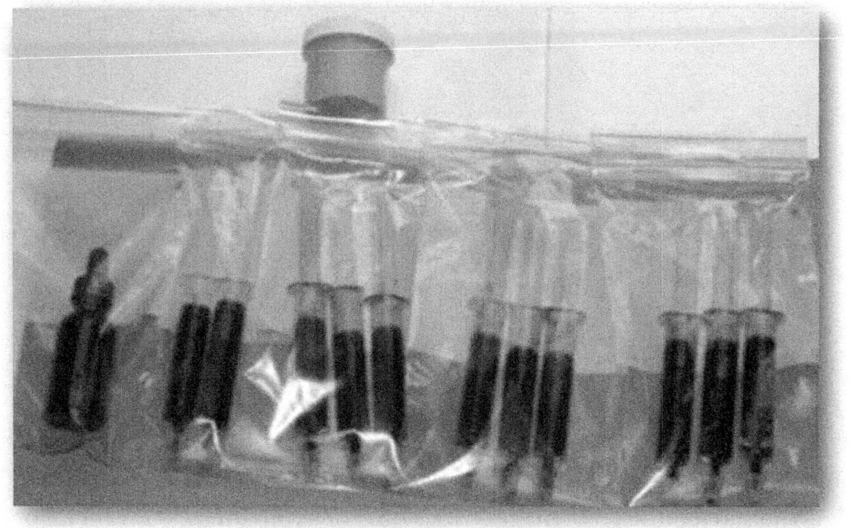

Ingredients for the SHORAK Protocol

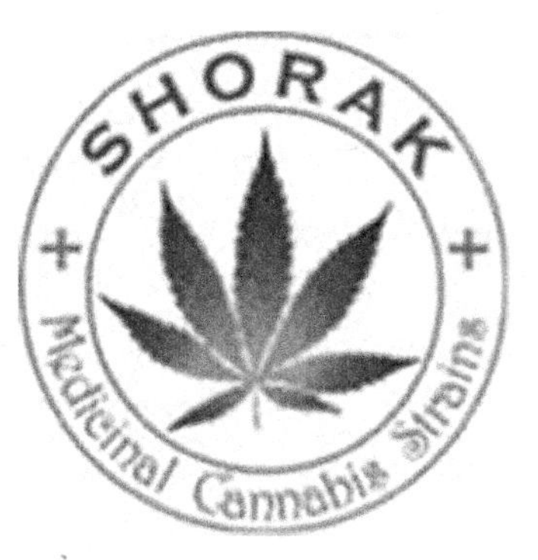

Mike Karohs
shorakoil@icloud.com

(This is the end of the SHORAK Cannabis Treatment Protocol.)

WHAT IF ONE ROUND OF TREATMENT IS NOT ENOUGH?

Most patients are cured after one round of cannabis treatment. If that happens to you, that is great! Congratulations! You have succeeded, and the oil has produced the results you hoped for. In that case it is advisable that you stay on the post- maintenance dose of approximately one gram of oil.

Some patients start using the oil only as a last resort after they have been treated (often repeatedly) with chemotherapy or radiation or—heaven beware!—both. The extent of damages caused by these treatments may be too great to be eradicated with one oil treatment. In that case, there are two possible scenarios: (1) Medical tests may show that the disease has been halted; it has not spread. Without the oil, the cancer would inevitably have metastasized and would have continued to spread. (2) So far, the cure has shown no effect. In both cases, don't despair! You have the weapon to kill the cancer, keep using it with faith! This is your only chance to defeat it.

Depending upon the extent of the damages that has been done, it may take as much as 180 grams of oil and up to six months to effectively kill the cancer. Even if your case is extremely serious, even in the terminal phase, remember that you are fighting for your life, the most precious gift you possess. Keep taking the oil until you succeed.

Helping friends

Once you start reaping the wonderful benefits of cannabis oil, you are most likely eager to share this amazing medicine with your friends. Few things are more heartwarming than helping someone who is desperate and hopeless. Each time it seems like a miracle when the oil cures one more patient who otherwise would be doomed to die.

Wrong assumptions

When I developed my sharing program I made a number of assumptions.

1. I assumed, that given the chance, everyone would be eager to be saved from a lingering and painful death. I was wrong. The truth of the matter is, there are people who simply *do not want* to heal.
2. I assumed that everyone really, desperately wants to live. I was wrong. There are people who simply *want* to die.
3. I assumed that people would be grateful for help and guidance in healing. I was wrong. As often as not, people tried to take advantage of me or even stab me in the back.

People who do not want to heal

There are truly people who do not want to heal. It seems there is a subconscious side to them that believes it may serve them better to hold on to their illness. While their conscious mind claims one thing, the subconscious mind says something else. This tendency is actually fairly common and is known as "psychological reversal." It is, in reality, a self-defeating strategy. Unfortunately, when psychological reversal is present, it will stop any attempt at healing dead in its track.

Folks with psychological reversal are actually easy to spot because most their answers will be followed by a limiting "but..."

I truly want to be cured, but...

... marijuana is illegal;
... if doctors thought it would work, they would use it;
... I did something bad in my past and don't deserve to be healed;
... my doctor does not approve of it;
... I want to finish chemotherapy first;
... I will lose my disability benefits;
... I won't get the attention (or sympathy) I crave;
... taking the oil would prevent me from driving;
... my wife (husband, children) will expect more of me when I am healthy;
... I may have to go back to that job I hate so much;
... the oil makes me feel "dumbed down";
... my doctor (family) would be mad at me
... it would be impossible for me to give up sugar.

(These are all authentic comments.)

One of the patients stopped the oil because she actually wanted her cancer to grow. Truly! She told us she was eating ice cream Sundays because sugar feeds cancer. Her reasoning was that if the cancer stopped growing she would not be admitted into a trial chemotherapy program. It seemed that she had feelings of unworthiness that were relieved by the extra attention she received from doctors and family, and from having large sums of money spent on her. She died 5 months into the trial.

People who do not want to live

And then, there are people who simply do not want to live. For some personal reason they wish to die. Their inner self seems to tell them that life just isn't worth living, and no medicine and no care can change this belief.

I particularly remember a fifty-eight year old woman with stage IV lung cancer. After the doctor gave her the diagnosis, she told her husband, "I am going home." Even though she underwent all the conventional treatments, she steadfastly maintained her stand. Her husband pleaded with her to take the oil, but she took it only very sporadically, just enough to help her with the pain. She died 3½ years after the first diagnosis. She seemed totally at peace and willing to "meet the Lord." It would not be how I feel, even though I really and sincerely respect this kind of faith.

People who take advantage of you

Most people I helped were grateful and thanked me with all their hearts. I have a large file of heartwarming "thank you" letters from people who have returned to full health after dosing themselves with the oil I provided to them.

> *From a patient:*
> *I will never be able to thank you, Mike, for all the wonderful things you've done in befriending me and giving me the affection, belief, advice, and the OILS!!! that you have spoiled me with. Frank*

However, there were also the folks who tried to take advantage of me. One couple comes to mind; the husband was diagnosed with colon cancer, and the wife was the caretaker. Within days after receiving the first syringe of oil, she called asking for another one because she allegedly was "out." This continued for weeks, with her calling every few days for more oil. Her excuses were, "I am out; it is not enough; this latest dose was too thin; I need more."(By the way, I never charged these folks as much as one cent. All my support was free, even though with all my medical bills I live on a very limited budget. This woman was very rich; yet expected me to give her "what she was entitled to"—her very own words.)

To make matters worse, the woman would not heed dosage instructions; she claimed that she had to "flood" her husband to get results (which is highly contra-indicated). She actually snatched another patient's syringe because she allegedly did not get enough. When she started using the oil for herself without getting a "card" (and refusing to get one), I had to cut her off. I was not going to get into legal troubles because of her.

Another patient, after accepting the oil, actually tried to tell negative things about me behind my back. His reasoning was that he wanted discourage others from using my oil in order to secure his own supply.

So if you are trying to help others, anticipate some disappointments along with the gratitude. Having saved yet another life from painful, heart wrenching death is well worth all the occasional disappointment.

What patients are writing

I have many, many letters from patients who were helped with SHORAK oil. But the most amazing is that of Stan.

Stan's story

When I first met 73-year old Stan, he had leukemia, lymphoma and colon cancer, COPD, emphysema, pneumonia, nearly incurable fungus, and A-fib. His doctors told him that he was incurable, but that they could keep him alive a little while longer with daily chemo pills—at $8000 per bottle for one month's supply. Stan and his wife were discussing the things she would have to handle after his death.

I initially provided SHORAK oil to ease Stan's final days, but to our greatest surprise, the story had an entirely different ending.

(Most of the letters below are from his wife Karen.)

12/17/14

Just wanted to say that Stan continues to show more baby steps improvement.
Things that I notice are ....he actually has recovery time now.
And he's continuing to get over his pneumonia.
He still gets very worn out, but he recovers now, and he is able to do more things.
It takes its toll, but he actually can get up and do more.

I think the cannabis oil is working and while it may be a little slow going, I'd hate to think where he would be without it, and I think he would most likely be in a heck of a lot more trouble.

12/19/14
Mike, I've seen the oil do soooooooooooooooooooooooo much for Stan's depression.
Which makes him want to do more. Yes he gets so very tired, but he does recover somewhat and somewhat quickly.
He's able to manage more.
And I think he's getting used to the oil too.
It's all making for a really nicer Xmas holiday, probably the best one we've had in a long time.

12/22/14
It was interesting, Stan and I had a conversation the other day, and I can tell the days when he takes less oil and the days he takes more. It is on the days with the oil that I see him as one of the nicest versions of Stan I've ever known. The difference in that alone is just uncanny and has made a gigantic difference and has made life vastly easier for his spouse. So I'm sure if its helping that much with the anger issues, to put it mildly...then if its doing even half as much for the cancer and lungs then Stan is tremendously blessed by your generosity.
He even looks different, because he is so much more relaxed.

12/23/14
I DO know Stan is blown away by your generosity and interest, and I know you have prolonged his life so that we can get things taken care of that we must, or things would have been left in a disaster, and I would have been left with a mess too big for my shoulders to carry.

12/24/14
But I am telling you…Stan spent the afternoon yesterday putting together some of the toys for the kids. He is doing more things like that since taking the oil.

12/24/14
Stan finally took my advice last night and took some SHORAK oil and so he said he slept really well!!
He says he still feels a little doped up. But I said it's probably because you took it with all your other sleeping pills. In any case, he's being just wonderful this morning.

12/30/14
There was a point a few short months ago where I was considering an anti-depressant. Things were unbelievably tough with Stan all last summer. Indescribable. SHORAK oil has made him into a kind and gentle man again.
There is a sweetness now that I'm grateful for that we can have our last remaining years together in peace and in harmony. For people who need an antidepressant, the oil is the only way to go. No harmful side effects; the only side effects are healing other internal areas in your body.
I call it my magic elixir.
P.S. On the day he had cut back on the oils he was being an old grump-ass again. When I suggested him putting the oil on the nerve pain from his torn rotator cuff he took my head off and wrote me a nasty note that he would not be putting any oil on him (cuz the smell I think). But when he was on the phone with his friend he shared with him that I feel he's so much easier to get along with when he takes the doses, and that I see finally a man I can co-exist with…well…he went back to taking the doses that soften the edges.
And life is quite different again (for me). Grateful.

01/08/15

Well I think we have good news.........!

Stan just got back from his appointment with the oncologist; looking over his blood test, and Stan told him about the SHORAK oil, and the doctor said whatever you are doing, keep doing it because while you'll always have the lymphoma and leukemia, it is being kept minimized and could be kept minimized for a long time. And things look good.

We also found out that 14% of the people who go on the chemo pills he is on, get pneumonia!?!

01/08/15

Anyway, people do not know what they are missing. SHORAK oil is such wonderful stuff. And I appreciate the calming effects it has too. I swear, its changed Stan's and my marriage. He is a changed man emotionally.

1/24/15

I wanted to jot off a note to you with some amazing news

All of Stan's blood tests now show that he is within tolerance levels (the parameters all show he is within the limits of tolerance)

When he got a Rife scan two days ago at the Naturopath's office, the difference blew our minds.

When he had the first Rife scan done about 15 months ago, it was 3 pages of gross maladies; and he had various cancer listed; at least 15 times cancer was showing up.

Guess what? When he had the Rife scan done just 2 days ago, cancer did not show up once!!

Not one time.

This time it was only one page of maladies, and it was almost alllllllll about the fungus.

He's still miserable from all of what is going on and so tired of the stuffed up head and constant runny nose and no energy ever..........but one thing at a time.
His oncologist knows he is taking the SHORAK oil, and he is duly impressed with how stabilized Stan's cancer has become. He said whatever you are doing, keep doing it!

01/30/15
The SHORAK oil is fantastic, and we feel like you are our guardian earth angel. I cannot believe that people are pussy footing around and not taking full advantage of your generous knowledge and gifts. You have given Stan and me much needed time and once he beats the remaining fungus, everything it will be better.

02/12/15
Stan's oncologist just reviewed his blood test, and Stan just called to tell me that his doctor said he is in Remission!!!! WOW. From Stage 4 lymphoma and leukemia!!!
I k.n.o.w it is the SHORAK oil you are providing us.
His lymph nodes are all back to normal size. The blood tests do not show the signs of the cancer anymore, they would have to do far more in depth testing to find it and where it stands. Amazing, Mike!!!!!
He still has terrible fatigue and the doctor said that is not due to the cancer but to all the other things going on with him.
Sometimes I think his fatigue is contagious. Just kidding.

3/1/15
It's been lovely to have the kind and good Stan back. Life is so much more harmonious. I think he has found his balance place with the oil.

3/26/15
I've not had a chance to get back with you........I think this is fantastic news below!!
You know how Stan was diagnosed with A-fib?
Well, he went to his oncologist last week, his oncologist took him OFF the Ibrutinib (chemo pills) saying they may be causing the A-Fib!
What a blessing in disguise.
I mean they see his blood tests are within normal ranges now, and they know the brutal side effects, so they have taken him off it. Why would he need it anymore in the first place? He didn't feel well for several days afterwards, and I said it was probably your body detoxing and getting used to being off of that awful nasty stuff.
And up until last week, he was to stay on those for the rest of his life. One wonders if they thought the "rest of his life" would not be so long.........

4/5/16
Stan is doing decent doses of the SHORAK oil, once in the morning and once at night. So I know he's just in an unbelievably better place than he was — the oil works so fast.
It's only been barely 5 months. All three cancers are gone and he is completely off chemo.
It's just amazing and I cannot fathom where Stan would have been if it weren't for SHORAK oil. I think life would have been very different. I feel you saved Stan's life. Because, like you said, once people get their 2nd round of chemo, it often lands them in hospice, and those chemo pills have some gnarly side effects.

4/8/15
Stan is taking his doses of oil. I think he knows it makes him more mellow and he is quite willing to do it. It's very good for our marriage. You should

market this to veterans with PTSD. I can testify to that beyond words. It has saved this marriage. The difference between Stan when he's on the right dose and when he's not is just profound.
He is a different person when he is on SHORAK oil.
It was a most unexpected side effect and gift in addition to what it did for his cancer.
To go from stage 4 lymphoma and leukemia to blood tests all within normal ranges, which I'm pretty darn sure is another way of saying he is in remission.....is just crazy.
His doctors act like the lymphoma will come back...but I told Stan, what do they know? With the SHORAK oil it may never come back! That is how I genuinely feel about it. And he agreed with me whole-heartedly.

4/20/15
I took Stan for a checkup last week. His neck is doing so much better since being on the cannabis oil that he no longer has to have shots for the pain caused from the accident from 3-4 years ago. I love seeing the expressions on the doctors' faces. The cancer remains in full remission.

5/7/15
I was so excited to drop a note off to you last night but had to wait until this morning.
Stan went to his kidney doctor yesterday, and the numbers are going in reverse now. Instead of getting worse, they are climbing back up in the right direction. Stan would be able to tell you specific numbers down to the decimal, and if low numbers are good or high or what, but I find it mildly confusing. For now, the main news, the simply great news is that his kidneys which were in grave trouble, and if they had gotten even the tiniest bit worse, he could have started into kidney failure and would have to look into dialysis, are now improving!! And the numbers are going in the opposite direction!!!

And all of his blood tests still show good/great news! All are still within normal range. I am simply amazed at the glorious wonders of the SHORAK oil.
He can now go out to lunch with his buddies, or out to dinner with me or his daughter and her family, and he has his own life here at home with computers, and he no longer has to have to get the shots of Botox into his neck from his neurologist. Most importantly, he is back to playing golf... his greatest regret when he thought he was dying was that he would never get to play golf again.

5/18/15
Stan was overwhelmed by your generosity. I would say flabbergasted and speechless by all the "gold" you gave us. He is just now getting everything stored and organized. If only you could have heard all the audible sounds we made as we opened the package, and Stan especially was astounded at much you supplied. He will really be set now. Thank you so much.
That ointment is a wonderful supplement. It helps so much with the pain from my ankle.

5/19/14
Letter from Stan:
I will get another CT scan in June, and that will tell me more as to the status of both the Chronic Lymphocytic Leukemia and the Small Lymphocytic Lymphoma – If I continue to remain stable and Lymph nodes are still normal size, I'm guessing I will be considered to be in full remission. Unbelievable.
Mike – The simplest I can say is you are an angel of mercy and sent to me by my Guides and a very evolved Guide and St. Germain. ***I guess God wants me to stay on this planet a little longer. It is so amazing the GOOD and Guidance you do.*** *What you gave us must be worth thousands of dollars plus the salves. I cannot estimate their worth.*

My oncologist does know I am on SHORAK oil and has no problem with that.
My love and blessings to you and I will keep you up to date.

According to a communication on 2/3/16, Stan is still in full remission. His emphysema, pneumonia, COPD, fungus and A-fib are also gone. In his own words, he is enjoying the life he never thought he would have again—while his wife is enjoying her kind and mellow husband.

What other patients are saying

(The following letters are from Andrea. She has pancreatic cancer and metastases all over her body.)

12/28/14
Dear Mike:
I am just back from the oncologist. It is unbelievable, but my blood markers are all in the normal range, and my liver values are also very good.
You don't know how thankful I am to you. Without you, I would no longer be alive. I am saying this with all my heart. You are my savior and my lifeline.
I am praying for you, and I hope you will not abandon me. Without you, I have no other options.
Thank you, thank you! Love, Andrea

01/16/15
The oil is my only salvation ....it is indeed salvation. I quite love it.

2/6/15
YES!! It was the SHORAK oil. It is so awesome I really love it. I've noticed it has eased some anxiety too, I feel much more relaxed and less anxious. So I am hooked. I love it more every day. Andrea

2/12/15
Dear Mike:
I have to share with you what I did with the infused ointment. I rubbed it underneath both my armpits because those lymph nodes were cancerous. Can you believe it, the lumps are getting smaller by the day, and the lumps on my liver are shrinking also. Love, Andrea

The last we heard from Andrea was that she had gained five pounds, and that she was going to get any further cannabis medication from close friends.

(Viola has bladder cancer that had spread all over her body.)

3/2/15
Dear Mike,
I went to the oncologist about two weeks ago and I was so weak my son practically had to carry me out of the car to sit in my chair to roll me into the doctor's office… I have had a huge turnaround in the last few days… since I started taking SHORAK oil.
Thank you with all my heart, Viola

3/15/15
May you, Mike, and your loved ones be well…I continue to be blessed with getting a bit better every day…I went to the oncologist on the 6th…I feel so wonderful that he has seen fit to keep me off chemo for four months

already…after the first surgery last year, I was in a chemo chair three days after I was out of the hospital! That's when he told me I would never be fully cured…and now they can no longer find the cancer.
Love. Viola

3/15/15
I am just so lucky and privileged, Mike, that you have become the Godsend that you are and a part of my healing process.
Viola

Letter from other cancer patients:

01/08/15
Feeling encouraged. What would we have done with out you.............I do not think we would be having this good news from the doctor, no I do not. What a gift you are.

01/25/15
Do please know that its simply fantastic, the results around the cancer so far. It is all stabilized, contained and seems to be neutralized. That is a blessing and relief. Regards, Matt

01/30/15
There is healing happening all over the place. Kathy

01/30/15
We are grateful, if it had been left up to us, we never would have could have grown it. This has been such a life-changing gift. You have truly extended Sam's life. There is no question. Love and blessings.

12/2/15
I went to Stanford for a checkup today. The big news is still no cancer! I believe that your oil is a big part of that. You have my admiration and thanks. Shirley

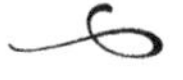

(The following letters are from Bill. He has chronic Inflammatory Demyelinating Polyneuropathy; he had colon cancer in 2003; in January 2015 doctor's suspected that colon cancer was returning.)

12/25/14
Your oils are so very amazing and I could never afford what you are giving me. Monetarily it is in the many thousands of dollars and the caring you send along with it is worth more than gold!!!!
I do believe the SHORAK oil and cannabinoids are very definitely helping me – I seem to have more energy and less fatigue. Bill

01/15/15
Bill's wife:
Just dropping by with a quick note.
Bill saw his kidney doctor yesterday and we had unexpected good news. His kidneys are holding their own and there was even a slight improvement. That was the area I was most concerned about.

01/25/15
Bill's wife:
Bill read your letters and commented on what completely kind and generous, caring person you are.
You have touched us both, separately and together. I keep my manual therapist abreast of what is going on and she is just flabbergasted at how much the oil has helped. She has witnessed it thru me.

01/28/15
My assessment of using SHORAK oil is very positive. It has definitely made internal improvements as my glucose is now in the correct range. I also believe it has effects on my PBH and overall I am feeling much better in general.
The ointment works very well on my hands and feet when they start getting painful. It certainly helps me get to sleep as the painful feet have kept me awake for hours. Bill

4/13/15
I received the package Saturday, thank you once again. I guess I have enough for some time as there were two vials, and it is noticeably stronger. I'll use it sparingly. The ointment seems to be doing a good job on my knees and shoulders. The pain has been reduced and I am able to stand much easier. That makes my life much better. The hands and feet still cause problems with sleeping. I don't know what I can do to relieve that pain. It seems very cyclic as I go days with little to no pain, then it comes back and lasts for two to four days.
Overall, I'm feeling better and it seems that my blood work is showing positive results in most areas, LDL, HDL, blood sugar etc. I still haven't got another test last Tuesday. Remember, the doctor spoke of the possibility of the colon cancer returning.
I truly appreciate your support for a complete stranger. Thank you. Sincerely, Bill

5/10/15
Dear Mike, I had a C-scan last week and it was good. There was nothing that showed any signs of cancer. I have one more test that will remove all doubt. I know it was the oil. I still have plenty of product to get me over these last hurdles.
I would like to express my great admiration for what you are doing. You are changing many lives for the better. I won't need the tube product, but I might want some of the ointment for future use. It does seem to provide

relief for the arthritic pain. I'll let you know in plenty of time when I need more. With lasting gratitude, Bill

5/27/15
Yes, I am still using the ointment and am finding good relief from arthritic pain. It does not seem to be as effective with the neuropathy pain, but it does seem to help most of the time. Bill
(I am preparing a stronger ointment for him, as his pain is unusually strong).

6/5/15
Remember, in January of 2015, my blood test showed renewed markers for colon cancer. After several months and many tests, it now has been definitely concluded that I no longer show signs of the cancer. That is certainly a relief. I'm so pleased and grateful that you were there to provide me with the best treatment I could get. Thank you so very much. I know it was the oil that helped me.
The stronger ointment seems to provide great relief to my knees and shoulders for the arthritic pain.
I will continue with SHORAK oil as I do believe it has helped my body over all. My HDL and LDL are in normal range, and it was very high before. My blood sugar levels have decreased to high normal, and in general my wellbeing seems to be much better now.
Again, I want to thank you for the wonderful treatment you have provided me. I could use a new supply in the near future when you have it available.
Sincerely, Bill

12/2/15
It has been a while since last we were in touch. You sent me great oil — again. The strength and make up were just right. I am in need of more now and hope to receive the same product.

The ointment is great too. This product certainly helps my over all well-being. I still have the neuropathic pain in my feet, most often at night. Taking this just prior to bedtime has allowed me to sleep in spite of the pain. The arthritic pain is managed well with the ointment on my knees shoulders and feet. I apply it generously after my shower to these areas and it helps a great deal. As that pain flares up during the day, I'll ply more of ointment as needed. All of this adds up to giving me a quality of life I would not have without this.

I just had a physical with my VA doctor and we discussed my use of this product. He is a non-believer in its cancer fighting ability. So again, I had an equivalent test to a colonoscopy — and again it showed I am cancer free. I know it is because of the oil.

Mike, I am still impressed with all you do and how you do it. I hope there is a special reward somewhere in your future for it.

Thanks again for everything.

Bill

The following letters are from Kris who was suffering from celiac disease and other intestinal problems.

12/25/14

I've had some growing digestion problems that have gotten increasingly uncomfortable the last several days. And nothing would bring down the tremendous bloat.

I'm telling you..........within minutes after taking the small amount in the eyedropper, I started to notice some ease in my tummy and it has continued. My tummy keeps feeling better and better and better. I'm thrilled.

Kris

12/30/14
I'm excited about and am in love with SHORAK oils. It only takes a very few short drops and I take them once in the morning and usually another very small dose in the evening. And it is keeping my tummy humming and you can physically see that my whole midriff area is no longer sticking out like it was.
I also appreciate how it has relaxed me, taken away an underlying angst.
Kris

12/30/14
The oil is still helping me so much. What its doing for my stomach is amazing. My gut is still healing up from the celiac disease and I don't know if I was getting IBS or what, but it was sheer misery the last few weeks.
I don't think a person truly "gets" just how amazing the oils are until it is actually experienced personally.
I am thinking of all my loved ones and wishing everyone had access to your genius. Maybe one day.........more people will, eh? Kris

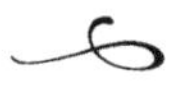

Letters from patients who use SHORAK oil for various purposes, like insomnia, high blood pressure, diabetes etc.

01/03/15
I do love leaving the infused oil out and letting it get so very soft. Makes it so easy to put on my ankle and then nibble on a little before bedtime. I did that last night and boy did I sleep!

01/03/15
Scott and I are extremely fortunate you chose to take us under your wings. You are our earth angels - we are blessed.

01/16/15

SHORAK oil is my only salvation ....it is indeed salvation. I quite love it.

02/6/15

I wanted to let you know that my most recent blood work numbers were great and I am cutting down and, will be stopping use of my anti anxiety med. I have been feeling wonderful. I can't thank you enough. My best to you, Nick

01/31/15

The oil infused with coconut oil really helped me finally get a full night's sleep last night!

I just needed to take a little bit more than usual. It used to take so very little but I've probably gotten used to it. I like eating it with the coconut oil.

And it's helping my digestion soooo much.

2/1/15

Yes agreed, the coconut infused oil tastes almost downright pleasant!! It's really helping me sleep to take some at night. Am thankful!

4/8/15

It's interesting about the blood pressure. Mine is lower since I have been using cannabis. I am sleeping better which is really good. Love, Ann

5/18/15

(Bobby started taking the oil for blood sugar/diabetes problems, he also has 4 stents in his heart, and he was forbidden to ride his Harley motorcycle for 5 years—he is a motorcycle repairman. After five months, his blood sugar levels are now normal, and he is allowed to ride his beloved Harley again).

Mike, this is wonderful oil you are providing me with, I love it! Bobby.

6/6/15
I started my cannabis treatments by smoking pot. I did not like it as it was very harsh on my throat. I tried other means of smoking using a pipe, a water filtered smoke, which was a bit better and finally a vaporizer which is the best method for smoking. But after I received SHORAK oil, I discontinued smoking.
I will continue with SHORAK oil as I do believe it has helped my body over all. My HDL and LDL are in normal range as it was very high. My blood sugar levels have decreased to high normal and in general my well-being seems to be much better now. William
I thank you for your kindness and generosity. I believe in what you are doing 100%. Thank you for helping so many people. Frank

How SHORAK cannabis strains were born

There are myriad marijuana strains available in dispensaries around the world. I have tried many of them, I have bred some of them and I have used them for vaporizing and oil making. There is no doubt that they work therapeutically. Still, the longer I worked with dispensary pot, the more there were things I didn't like. For example:

- The state does not impose standards for quality, safety or potency in the production of marijuana; and since dispensaries typically do not divulge the source of their marijuana, customers must rely on their word about plant quality, cannabinoid content, adherence to organic growing regulations, etc.
- Much of the dispensary pot has been crossbred back and forth for decades, which tends to degrade it.
- Many of the dispensary products are from plants that are only four to five months old. Using immature plants does not allow for the full development of the plant's medicinal potential.

Cancer is a devastating disease that kills without mercy. For that reason, I wanted strains that kill cancer with a vengeance, strains that

- have top quality genetics;
- originate from the highest quality landrace strains;

- are potent cancer killers;
- are anti-inflammatory;
- address lack of appetite;
- soothe anxiety and keep insomnia at bay;
- boost the immune system;
- are gentle on the body without negative side effects.

But I simply could not find strains like that at the dispensaries. So the only solution was growing my own.

And that is how SHORAK cannabis strains were born.

In the beautiful Cachagua region near Big Sur in California, I have bred or developed dozens of medical strains, mostly for the treatment of various cancers, but also for other serious diseases like epilepsy, autism, Parkinson's disease, MS, pain management, insomnia, etc. (I sincerely hope that further legalization will soon make it possible for me to share these with patients around the world.)

While pot shops around the worlds are selling knockoffs or mixes of the myriad of dispensary strains with goofy names, I did something entirely different.

Growing medical Cannabis is not simply a matter of getting a few seeds from different countries and dropping them into the soil. Producing superior phenotypes requires growing numerous sample plants from specific landrace strains and examining them for just the right genetics. I used this important first step to find the perfect individuals to crossbreed together.

I then used seeds from the crossbred plants and backcrossed those with each other to create stabilized strains.

After these stabilized strains were grown, I selected the best individuals from the offspring.

I then put these chosen individuals through a very important rejuvenation process. This means letting each plant root and grow many green shoots, which are cut off and dipped in a rooting solution.

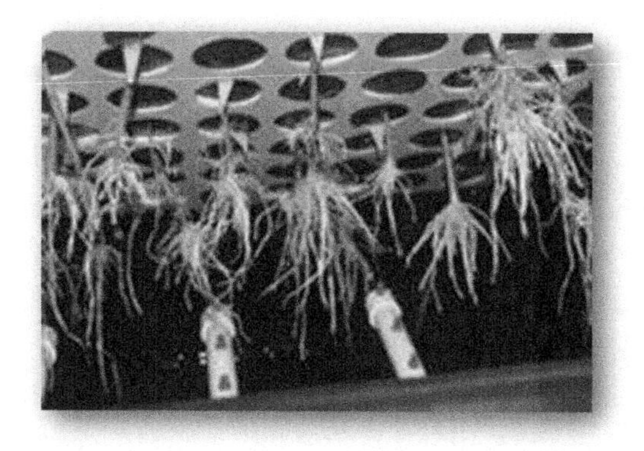

The resulting clones are allowed to grow for several weeks. Before they are flowered out, more clones are taken from them.

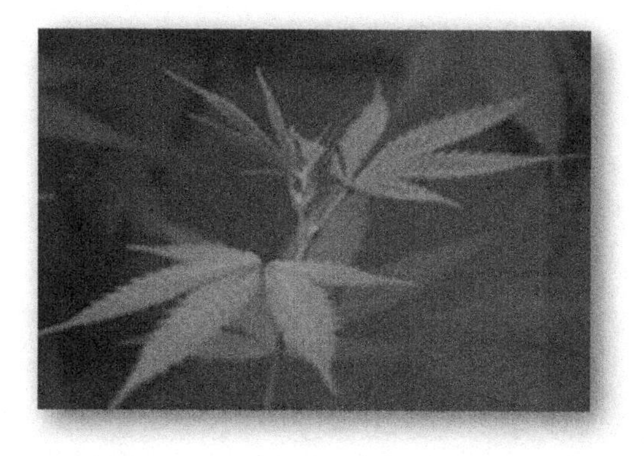

The strongest cannabis strains are found in warm countries where the growing season can be as long as ten or eleven months. I imitate this lengthy growing process by aging the clones. Experience has shown that clones retain the age of the original plant. Including the clone-aging cycle allows plants to develop their full medicinal potential.

Once clones get past the age of seven or eight months, they are considered fully developed. From then on, more clones may be cut from clones indefinitely without any deterioration of the plant or genetic drift. Clones will remain perfect as long as they are grown under ideal growing conditions. All of my clones are cultivated under very stringent conditions. They are also grown under the highest quality professional grow lights or natural sunlight, if possible.

For fertilizing I use only 100% organically certified plant foods and micronutrients, and the plants are watered with reverse osmosis filtered water.

Before full maturation, all my plants go through an extensive 3-week flushing process to ensure that there is absolutely no fertilizer residue or anything else impure in the final product.

Admittedly, the breeding, the selection procedure, the back crossing, the clone aging, and the extensive flushing seems like a lengthy process, but it is only by following each individual step that I am able to create these exceptional cannabis strains with the most potent and powerful medicinal properties.

Senior strain.

My first low THC/high CBD strain became quickly known as the SHORAK *Senior strain* for very obvious reasons.

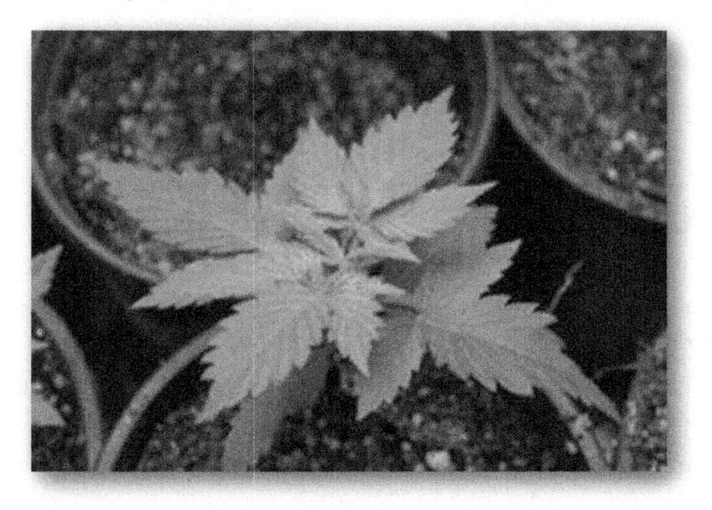

The overall effect is very mild. It is low in THC and medium high in CBD. Even elderly, very sick, and/or medically fragile patients can use it with the minimum psychoactive effect while at the same time obtaining the highest possible therapeutic benefits.

The higher CBD level is very significant. In addition to possessing an incredibly wide range of medicinal properties, it is non-psychoactive. In fact, it diminishes the psychoactive effect of the THC. The presence of CBD with THC often reduces the feelings of anxiety that some people feel with higher levels of THC.

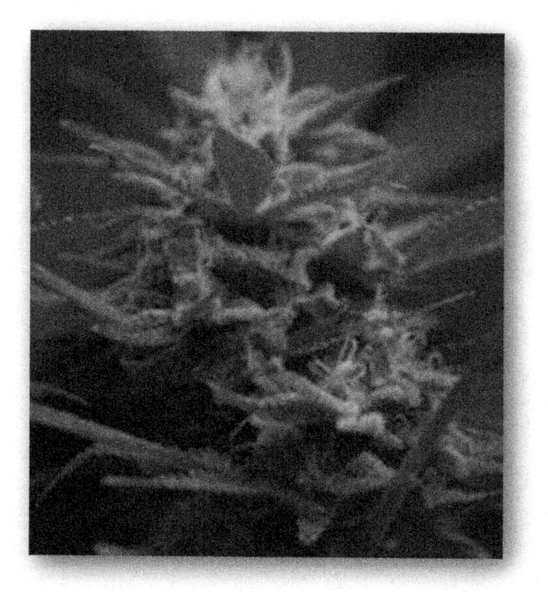

The CBD in the *Senior* strain is derived from tropical sativa, rather than from indica strains. Sativa strains are fundamentally of higher quality because they were bred to be of smoking quality. The addition of the tropical Sativa strain gives *Senior* its mildness.

The *Senior* strain would be excellent for patients trying Cannabis treatment for the very first time.

The *Senior* strain is ideal for diluting stronger strains. For instance, brain or lung cancer patients require strains with a higher THC content; the *Senior* strain can be added to the high THC strain to adjust the THC level up or down.

Because of its high CBD content, the *Senior* strain also seems to be a strong preventative for the onset of chemotherapy-induced neuropathy, a side effect of some chemotherapy drugs. Equally important, it is an excellent strain to produce oil with a mild effect.

Under the strict supervision of a doctor I feel that this strain may be mild enough to be used for children.

Senior Ultra strain

This hybrid is a combination of a Ruderalis and a medium level THC sativa strain. (The picture shows a batch of freshly made Senior Ultra oil.)

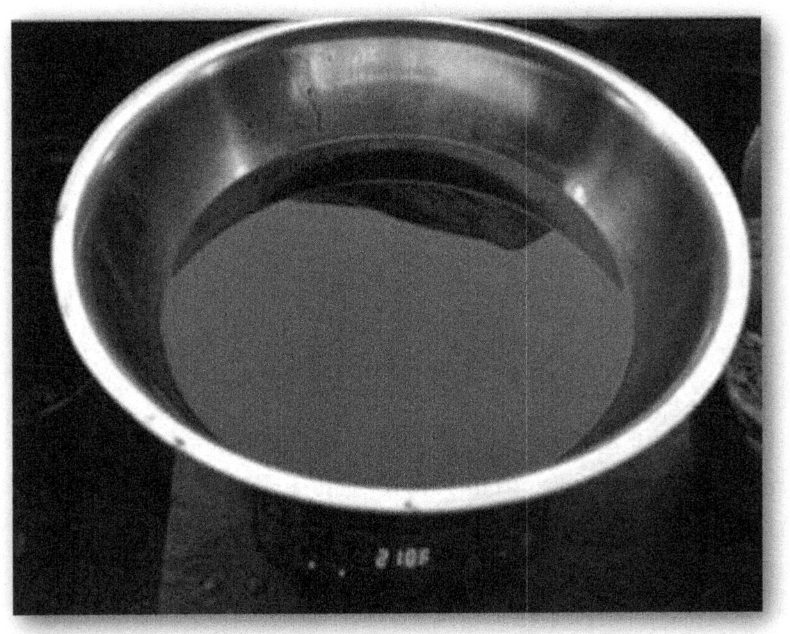

Freshly made Senior Ultra oil

Because it has a slightly higher THC and much higher CBD content than the *Senior* it has the potential to be used for many medical purposes.

It is stronger than the *Senior* and was developed specifically to be made into oil.

#2037 Afghan hybrid

I developed this strain for more experienced cannabis users in our patient support group. It has numerous therapeutic qualities. With higher THC level and moderate CBD levels, this strain works well for cancer treatment requiring a combination of both these cannabinoids. #2037 also works well for stress, insomnia, muscle spasm, pain, eating disorders and asthma.

This strain is suited especially well as basis for oil; but should only be prescribed for someone who does not mind some psychoactive effect.

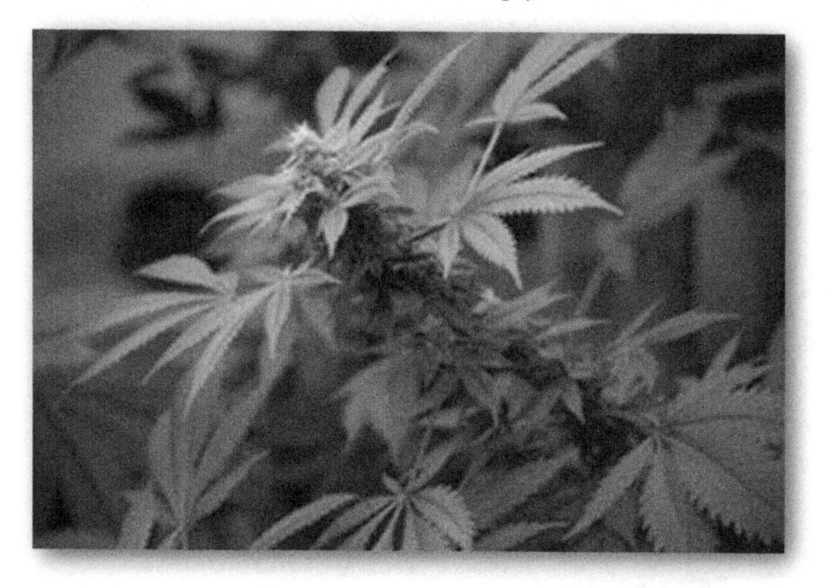

African Swazi

This is a somewhat domesticated strain from Africa. Native people have used it for hundreds of years. This strain has the typical strength for which many of the African strains are known.

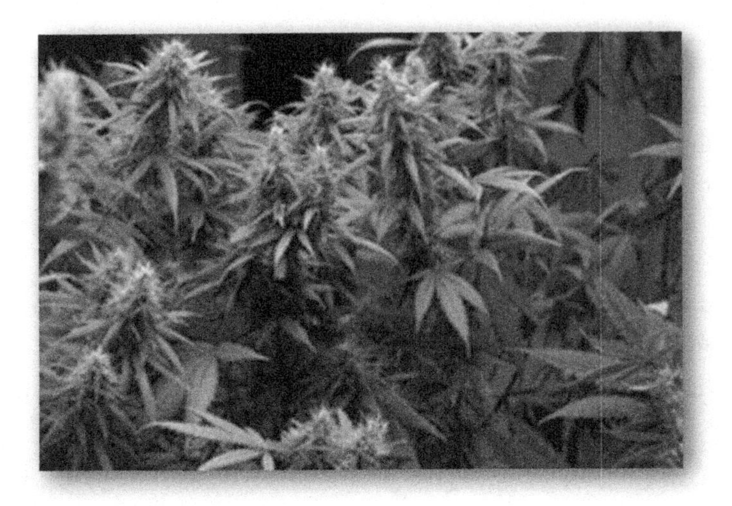

The plant is of special interest because it is extremely high in THCv, which is known to be effective for diabetes, epilepsy, and seizures.

Black Afghan/Mazar

This is a hybrid between a Black Afghan and a Mazar. Mazar is considered to be one of the highest quality Indicas in the world, and Black Afghan is know for having numerous medicinal qualities.

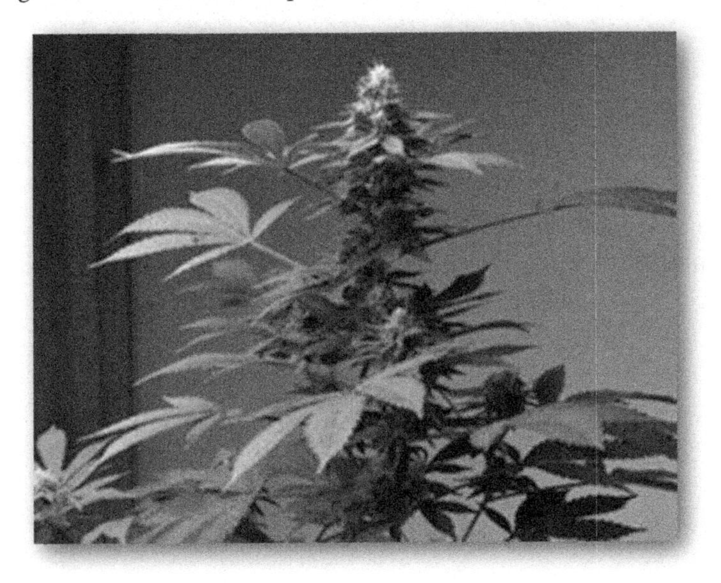

With its higher CBD levels it is useful for people with pain management issues. It has been used for depression, stress, insomnia, muscle spasms, pain, asthma and eating disorders. It works well for increasing patients' appetites.

The hybrid has a THC level of about 20% and CBD of about 4 to 5%.

This strain is an especially good basis for oil, and it is also well suited for someone who does not mind the psychoactive effect.

Koh-Chang Thai

Very knowledgeable growers have cultivated this Asian cannabis for thousands of years and have created very sophisticated genetics.

Koh-Chang Thai is a species with a great potential for patients needing extremely high quality THC. Its CBD content is between 1 and 2%.

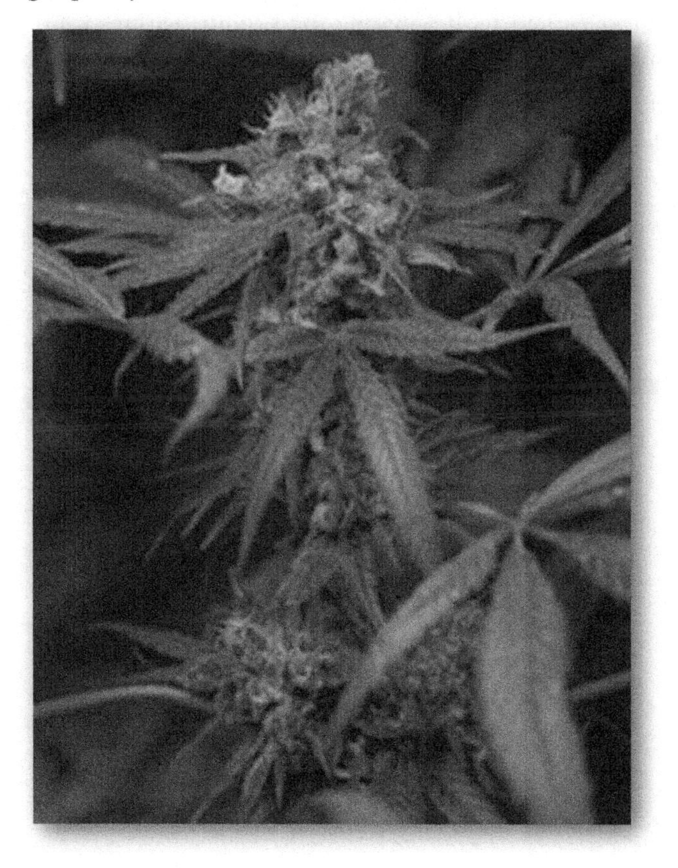

#2017 RS-strain (original)

I developed this strain for two purposes:

1. To create a superior general-purpose medicinal strain for a wide range of uses.
2. To demonstrate the results of combining only the finest cannabis genetics available.

For this strain I started with the two highest quality medicinal sativas available and crossed them with each other. I selected two of the most promising offspring and crossed those with one of my high CBD ruderalis mother strains.

#2017 exceeded even my own expectations for cancer treatment. It cured a breast cancer patient with a marble-sized tumor within 5 months without chemotherapy, radiation, or other conventional treatment.

Additionally, this strain helps greatly with mood enhancement and pain relief. It also works well for severe cases of insomnia.

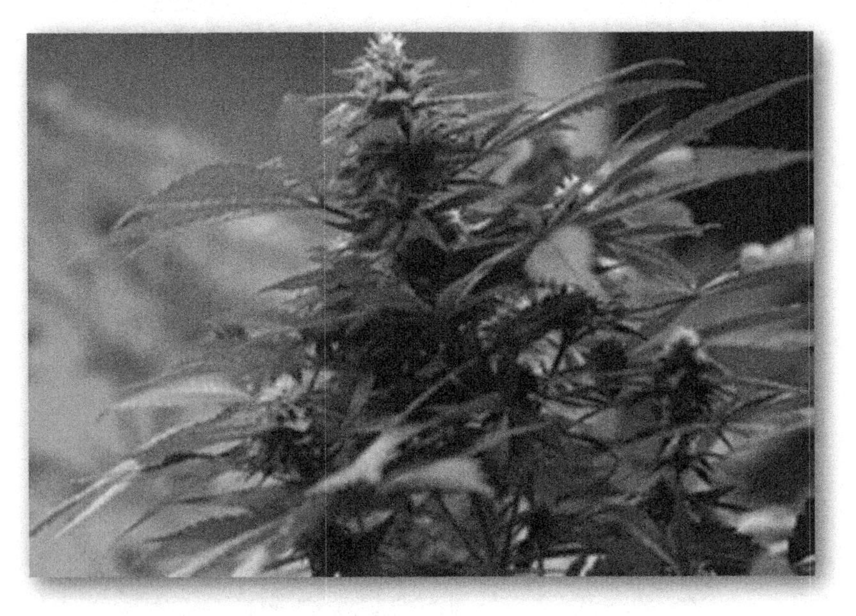

Since the original RS strain proved so successful I decided to develop several more high CBD variations and also several high CBD/THC strains for specific medicinal purposes.

RS-31 strain

The RS-31 strain is one of the varieties with a higher THC content. It is intended for patients with illnesses needing both the CBD and THC effect. I achieved the effect by combining the original stabilized RS 2017 strain with a Nepalese variety, which can reach THC levels of up to 28%.

Making the RS 31 strain into a four-way hybrid also increased the terpene spectrum, which further enhanced its medicinal benefits.

RS-37 strain

The effectiveness of the original RS strain compelled me to create a hybrid strictly for oil production. I started with two of my most medicinally potent indicas, (which I already had used successfully for oil making) and crossed them with the original RS-2017. The resulting RS-37not only retained the high quality sativa influence of the original RS-2017; the addition of the two indica hybrids resulted in an amazingly powerful multi-strain variety for making oil.

RS-40 strain

RS-40 is another strain intended for making oil. This time, I started with high CBD ruderalis and crossed it with an indica hybrid. Adding a high THC Nepalese strain enabled me to create a high CBD/THC strain for patients needing this particular medication.

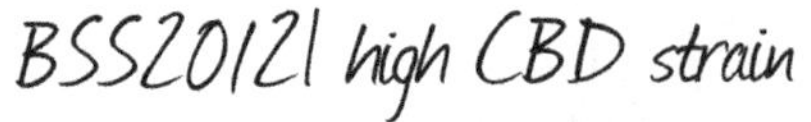

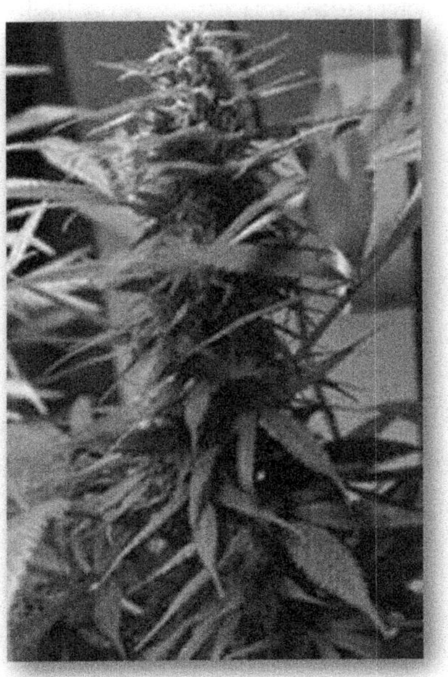

For BSS20/21, I crossed two well-known CBD strains which are recognized for their anti-seizure properties. From their offspring I selected the most promising individuals. To increase CBD levels even further, I crossed these offspring with one of my own high-CBD strains.

Because of its remarkably strong anti-convulsant properties, this high-CBD three-way hybrid is ideally suited for patients with seizures or epilepsy.

This strain is also suitable for many purposes where high-CBD cannabis is advisable.

Elephant oil

This is a very special oil strain that got its whimsical name from Dave, a patient who said, "This oil is strong enough for elephants, it knocks me right over."

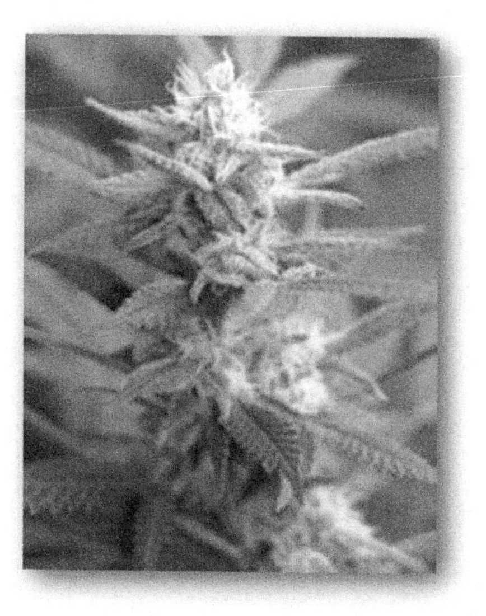

I actually created the strain specifically for Dave who was in extremely poor condition when we met for the first time. He had stage-4 colon cancer, and doctors had told him that there was nothing more they could do for him. They said that at the most he had five months to live.

Dave had just completed another round of chemotherapy and was in so much pain that even with a "donut" pillow he was unable to sit. After 5 weeks of oil therapy, Dave was starting to feel better. His cancer went into remission and he was able to go for long walks with his dog along the beach.

And then, unfortunately, there were complications due to earlier surgery, and Dave had to return to the hospital. For several months, he was off the oil, and the cancer returned with a vengeance. More chemotherapy was prescribed with the result that the cancer was metastasizing all over Dave's body, including his liver.

Dave was now in worse shape than when we met originally. That's when I decided to create Dave's special oil.

To make it super-strong, I crossed several of my heaviest indica strains with one of my highest CBD plants. The results were exactly as I had anticipated. After starting the oil, Dave said that other patients should be warned of the severe "couch lock effect." He said that after taking a dose all he wanted to do is sit.

For Dave's cancer, the elephant oil worked incredibly well. He is again in remission. His cancers are shrinking, and finally, he is on the road to recovery. A few weeks ago, he bought a new motor home and is planning a vacation trip with his family.

CBD-OD

A ruderalis strain crossed with a Nepalese plant has resulted in this hybrid with potentially 10 to 20% THC and high CBD.

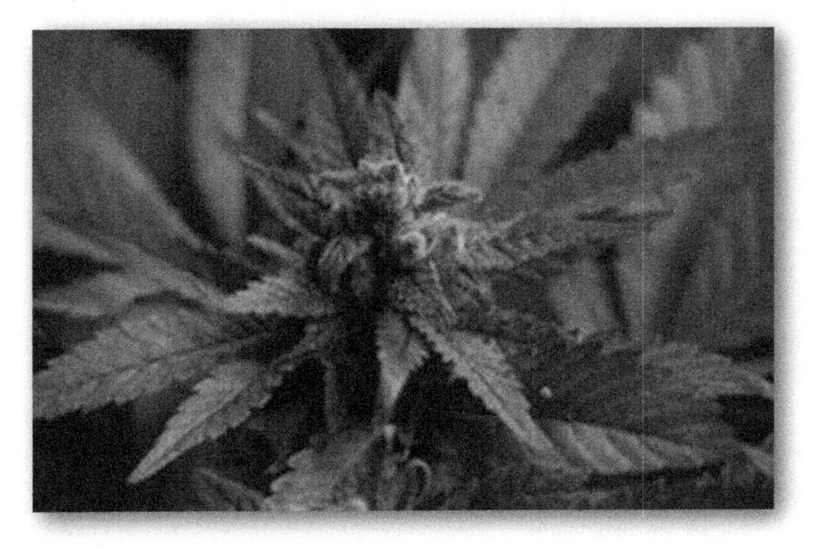

Under a doctor's supervision, this would be a devastating cancer killer. It would be an excellent strain for all kinds of cancer and other illnesses needing high THC and CBD content.

Black Durban

Black Durban is one of the finest sativas I have ever seen, although I am not certain exactly where in Africa it originated. It looks like the type of sativa that is found in rare locations in high mountain valleys. It is clearly not the kind of commercial Durban that is often found on the streets of Europe.

The plants are tall and slender with extremely dark, large leaves, and they produce the classic and very beautiful long cone buds typical of Durban. They still retain the wonderful flavor of their long-distant Asian ancestors.

Black Durban has proven to be very suitable for a wide range of medicinal uses, especially where high quality THC is required. It is also an excellent strain for making indica/sativa hybrids. In my opinion this could easily someday become a major-league commercial strain, as famous as Blue Dream, or White Widow, or OG Kush, or some of the other legendary strains.

Durban-el

I don't know how to speak any of the African languages; but a friend who gifted me with this rare strain says that the "el" is vernacular meaning "genuine, "or "authentic or "the real thing." He said that according to the locals, this plant has been grown in small plots for their personal use as far back as their forefathers can remember.

This plant is somewhat perplexing. It is bushier and leafier than any of the Durban strains I know. It grows the classic cone-shape Durban buds, but they are very thick and resinous and almost resemble an indica or an indica hybrid. Nevertheless, it is a wonderfully healing plant and whatever it is, I love it.

Durban-el is fragrant and delicious and has a THC level in the low to mid 20%.

When grown in the inland valleys of California, this becomes some of the finest cannabis I have ever seen.

Durban-el is ideal for anyone needing a high quality THC strain.

Durban-Oaxan

This cross between two very popular and very high quality sativas was originally developed as a dispensary strain. Interestingly, it has been found to have significant mood enhancing properties and gives users a strong overall sense of wellbeing. While its other medicinal effects are not as strong as those of other species, it should work well for patients wanting to smoke or vaporize Cannabis for depression or mood enhancement.

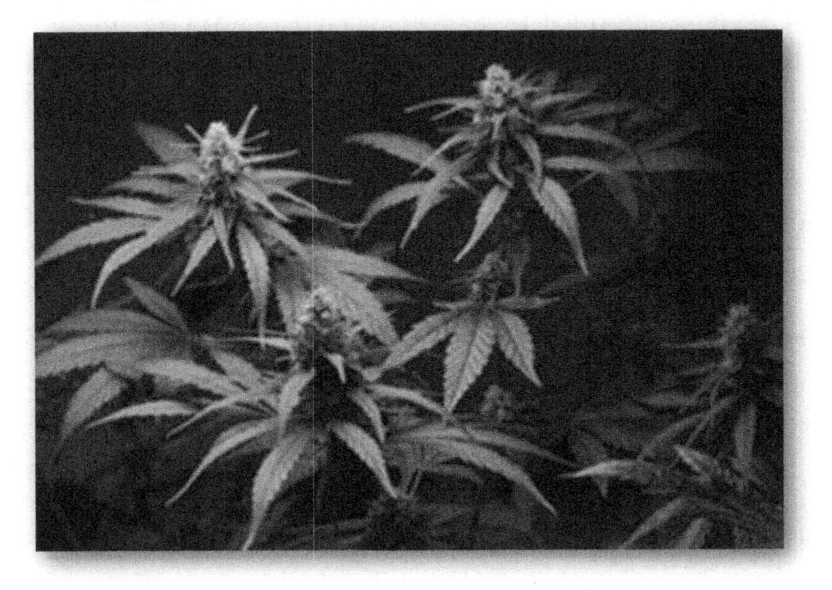

Brazilian White

This indica/sativa hybrid is a cross between a Brazilian White strain and a Nepalese indica. It has exceptionally valuable genetics and can reach THC levels of up to 28%.

This strain has the therapeutic potential for relieving depression and anxiety: it can ease sleep disorders caused by autoimmune diseases, and it may alleviate Restless Legs Syndrome (RLS).

The oil made from this hybrid has the potential to alleviate pain for cancer patients.

It likely would be a very effective medication for lung cancer, brain cancer, lymphoma and other illnesses requiring a higher level of THC.

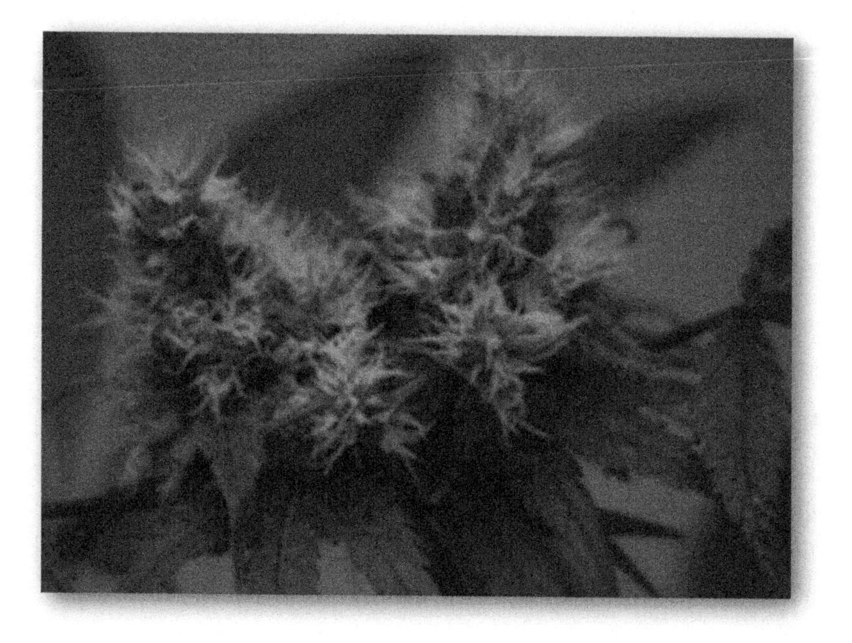

The higher THC level offers a greater latitude to titrate THC up or down by adding a weaker strain such as *Senior*.

Oaxacan-Congolese

I bred the Mexican Oaxacan because we like this particular variety for its mildness; yet it is still very potent.

It was originally an experimental hybrid, which turned out to be very popular and suitable for making edibles. People who consume them claim it makes them feel very happy and kind of dreamy and in a very good mood.

The Oaxacan is known for its mood enhancing properties.

SHORAK STRAINS ARE MULTI-PURPOSE

All my strains are well suited for smoking, vaporizing, or other ways of consumption; but most of all, they are ideally suited for making oil, which I still consider the most powerful way to administer cannabis medicine. The results are proving my assumptions. Patients testimonials and letters keep telling me about their effectiveness.

From a patient:
Stan's oncologist just reviewed his blood test, and Stan called to tell me that his doctor said he is in Remission!!!! WOW. From Stage 4 lymphoma and leukemia with SHORAK oil!!!

From a patient:
To us both, its high, high, high praises to the blessed SHORAK oil. Stan and Karen

Introducing SHORAK seeds

An added benefit from developing SHORAK strains are seeds. After developing each strain into a genetically stabilized version, storing the seeds in my seed bank now enables me to reproduce identical copies of all these wonderful strains I created as often as needed.

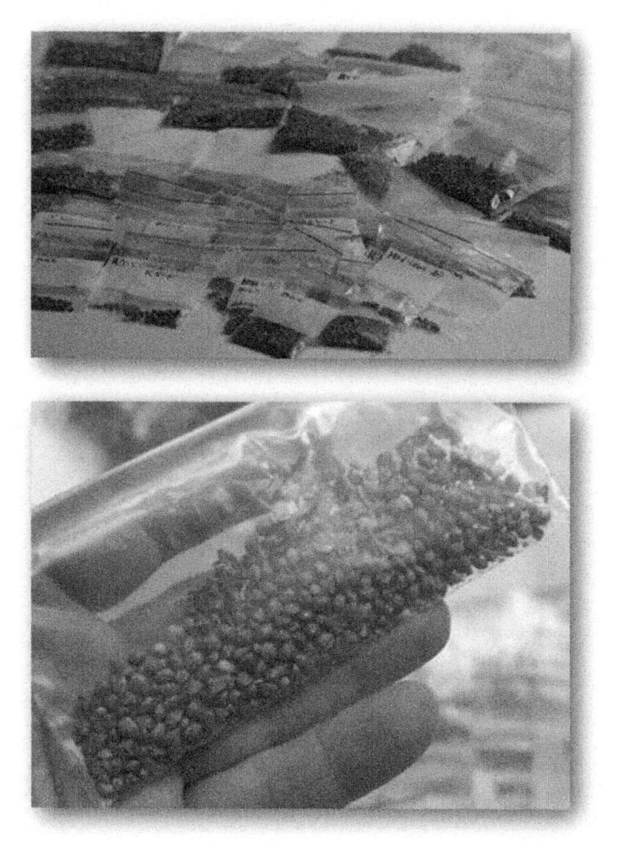

It has been long road, and often a difficult one. There were successes and setbacks. But I prevailed. My future plans involve matching specific cannabis strains to individual patients and/or diseases. Most of all I hope that with further legalization SHORAK strains and seeds can be made available to patients and doctors on a much greater level, perhaps even around the world.

Conclusion

I wrote this book so you and your loved ones can benefit from my experience. I encourage you to use this new knowledge to forge your own path toward healing. Determine that you will not be another fatality of the drug industry. Fight for your right to live, and treat yourself with medicines that work. Cannabis has curative qualities that seem almost miraculous.

As I mentioned in the Foreword, (I am repeating it here in case you normally do not read Forewords) once you start this program do not stop halfway. If you do, the cancer that seems defeated, will double its strength and return with greater vehemence.

After being in temporary remission, Jane, a lung cancer patient, stopped the oil midway. Instead, she decided to participate in a six-year chemotherapy trial, which promised more attention from doctors and family than taking the oil. About six weeks into the trial, doctors told her that she had to quit; the chemotherapy was enhancing her cancer and actually made it grow and metastasize. Jane died only a few months later.

The treatment has to continue until the patient is fully cured. To monitor results, patients need to stay in the care of doctors and undergo regular tests and examinations by specialists.

Even after you are completely cured and go back to your normal life, there should be tests periodically by qualified health practitioners to confirm that your remaining in sound health.

Cannabis has worked a miracle in my own life; it has worked for my friends and for patients in our cancer support group. I hope that this book will inspire you to take charge of your own health, too. Defeating cancer is your own fight. You cannot rely on doctors to cure you. There are many good doctors, but unfortunately, there are also those who will only try to prolong patients' life as long as possible, so that they can suck as much money as possible out of them before they die.

If through my book I can save other cancer patients from dying needlessly, my purpose will be fulfilled.

My warmest wishes for your health and healing.

Acknowledgements

Before signing off, I want to say special thanks my mother, Dr. Erika Margarethe Karohs, who helped me write and turn this book around in record time. Without her, it would not have been written.

Incidentally, she was also the caretaker during my battle with cancer—and she is truly the world's greatest mother, second to none. I would not have survived cancer without her. I thank her with all my heart.

Thanks also to my friends and patients at the Cancer Center who used SHORAK oil to cure themselves and supported me with their encouragement and feedback.

Last, but not least, my special thanks to you, gentle readers, for buying this book. I hope that it is helping you to more fully understand the amazing healing that cancer patients can achieve with cannabis.

Finally, if you find my book helpful to you or one of your loved ones, please leave a review on Amazon. Please do it now, it will only take a few minutes of your time, otherwise, you might forget. Thank you very much.

Mike Karohs

shorakoil@icloud.com

Made in the USA
Las Vegas, NV
03 February 2021

17006427R00075